Dedication

To Laurie—
who paddled the front cockpit, braved the bears,
pointed out the beauty, and did the initial editing
of this book.

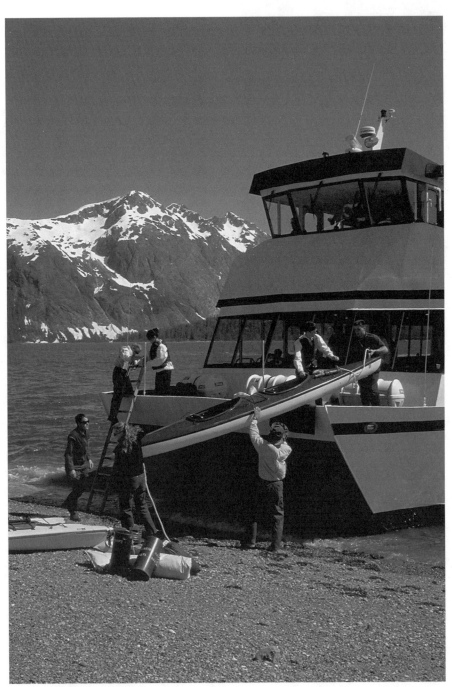

Tour boat dropping off kayakers

Adventure Kayaking
Trips in Glacier Bay

Don Skillman

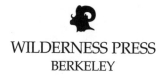

WILDERNESS PRESS
BERKELEY

Library of Congress Card Number 98-19151
ISBN 0-89997-225-X

Manufactured in the United States of America
Published by: Wilderness Press
2440 Bancroft Way
Berkeley, CA 94704
(800) 443-7227; FAX (510) 548-1355
mail@wildernesspress.com
Contact us for free catalog
Visit our web site at www.wildernesspress.com

Front cover: The west side of Muir Inlet, below Hunter Cove, looking across to Muir Point, with Mt. Wright in the distance.

Back cover: *top:* Gray wolf
bottom: Icebergs in Muir Inlet

Library of Congress Cataloging-in-Publication Data

Skillman, Don.
    Adventure kayaking : trips in Glacier Bay / Don Skillman. — 1st ed.
        p.   cm.
    Includes bibliographical references (p.   ) and index.
    ISBN 0-89997-225-X (alk. paper)
    1. Sea kayaking—Alaska—Glacier Bay National Park and Preserve.
    2. Glacier Bay National Park and Preserve (Alaska)—Guidebooks.
    I. Title.
    GV776.A62G537   1998
    797.1'224798'2—dc21
                                                                98-19151
                                                                CIP

Table of Contents

Introduction

"And then the ice came. It was
not just a white dot in the
distance. It came fast. It
knocked down all the houses.
The people had to leave."

—*from a Chookenaidi oral history*
of their fleeing before advancing
glaciers at the beginning of the
Little Ice Age, 4000 years ago.

The Chookenaidi, a sub-tribe of the Tlingits who inhabited Southeast Alaska, did indeed flee Glacier Bay, with advancing glaciers at their heels. Huge glaciers covered the bay for many centuries. Forests that had existed there were partly sheared off, partly buried, or completely scraped away. The landscape was altered in ways that only relentless glaciation can perform. Then, for no apparent reason, the glaciers receded as quickly as they had advanced. But the native people did not recolonize Glacier Bay. They founded a new village at Hoonah, on Chicagof Island, some thirty miles from the mouth of Glacier Bay. Hoonah is the home of many descendants of this tribe today.

Today, a portion of Glacier Bay is still locked beneath glaciers. As for the remainder, the fiords and land are renovated and newly released. The story is there in the water, the ice, the rock, and the plants. You too can read it.

*   *   *   *

Ever wish you could kayak in a wilderness so astounding, so remote and unspoiled, that you would be constantly inspired by its magnificence? The scenery would dumbfound you; the isolation awaken a spirit that lies suffocating in most of us. You can do just that. This book will tell you how and where.

Imagine a narrow bay, a twisting fiord 65 miles long, locked under the glacial ice flow—a slow-motion river of ice some 4000 feet thick—that is carving it. The ice flow has exerted up to five million tons of pressure over each acre for millenniums as it crushes and grinds inexorably at bedrock, inching along to the seduction of gravity. Only the highest peaks surrounding the fiord jut from the creeping ice monster; the bay, its islands, and streams are invisible and inaccessible, locked beneath a frozen shroud.

Now imagine a relatively rapid melting, as perhaps simulated with time-lapse photography, where 65 miles of the captive bay emerges from the ice age. The elapsed time is not thousands of years, but a mere two hundred—

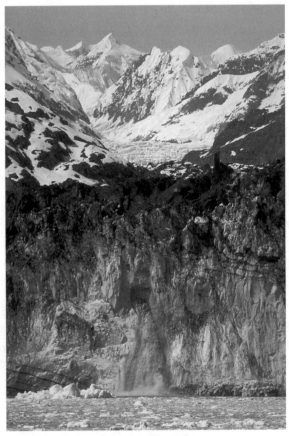

Margerie Glacier calving into Tarr Inlet

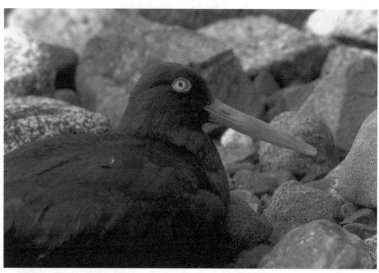

Curious black oystercatcher

hardly equal to three human lifetimes. Meltback at this rapid rate is unprecedented in history. Yet this is what happened at Glacier Bay, 60 miles west of Juneau in Southeast Alaska.

These events have created an astonishing landscape. Deep, blue-water fiords provide the paddler a highway, bordered by shorelines which can slope steeply upward until frosted thousands of feet above by perennial snowfields. The bay is cradled by snowcapped peaks, the loftiest being 15,320' Mount Fairweather to the west. Glaciers either creep slowly into tidewater, or their snouts are nearby, filling newly-carved valleys. Glacial streams pour in meltwater thick with silt and glacial flour.

From the paddler's perspective the geographic vastness is more than impressive; it's almost overwhelming. Three mountain ranges, split by the extensive fiord system that is Glacier Bay, present a magnitude that dwarfs the kayaker. You get to view this grandeur, while rocking gently in your kayak among bergs calved from the glacial face before you. But words, alone, won't do; you have to see it for yourself. This book helps you do just that.

Though the bay is truly a wilderness, you won't be alone. Several thousand seals visit here in spring and summer to calve on ice floes near the head of inlets. Lucky paddlers will see humpback whales that arrive in June breaching or feeding. You may spot the dorsal fins of orcas, or the surfacing apogees of cavorting porpoises as they breathe explosively. This book describes where whales and seals are most often seen. Birders are in ecstasy too. Tufted puffins, phalaropes, cormorants, oystercatchers, ducks, gulls, many shorebirds, and eagles are common. Your kayak is ideal for approaching silently and slowly, enjoying good viewing without getting so close that the birds are alarmed. Both brown bears and black bears patrol along the shoreline. Wolves may howl at night, or even during daylight hours. Scan the higher slopes for mountain goats, and near the shoreline for moose.

While there are nearly mature forests near the mouth of the bay, as you paddle north the trees become younger and shorter. Near the north end of the bay plant communities are made up of willow, alder, and cottonwood, with few conifers. Near the glaciers, only a few mosses, dryas and forbs struggle to gain hold. Recently uncovered rock and till support no plant life at all. Visiting here is a journey back to the ice age.

The bay is a natural laboratory, offering easily read, graphic displays of both glaciation and plant succession. How do forests become established? How long before fish inhabit streams newly uncovered from glacial ice? As new lands are freed from the ice, how much time must pass before those areas are utilized by the various plants, birds and animals which will inhabit them? This book pinpoints the places where you can see the answers yourself.

There are few time machines like Glacier Bay. Here the melting of tidewater glaciers, following their own mysterious cycle unrelated to short-term climate change, has compressed time. The aura of the effects created so clearly here, where the paddler can breathe spruce-scented air in one place, and the acrid odor of newly uncovered rock in another, cannot be dismissed; it is primal in nature.

This book is not only for the expedition kayaker. Much of Glacier Bay is protected water feasible for the beginner. Several areas offer motorless seclusion in a labyrinth of channels ideal for shorter trips. Organized trips are another way of experiencing Glacier Bay from the paddler's perspective.

This book is intended to inform you of what is there, to guide you to it, and to add to your overall Glacier Bay experience. Equipment and safety are discussed, but this is not primarily a how-to-kayak book. It is a guide that will help you enjoy the powerful thrills to the senses that await in this magnificent country. Once you experience Glacier Bay from a kayak, you will be changed for life.

Chapter 1

About Glacier Bay

Geography and History

Beginning at the south end of Vancouver Island, the Pacific Coast of British Columbia and Southeast Alaska are protected for 900 miles by the long arc of an island chain. These protected waters are the famed Inside Passage. The northern end of Alaska's Inside Passage is at Cross Sound, 70 miles west of Juneau. From this point northward, the Alaska coastline is exposed to the open-sea conditions of the Pacific and the Gulf of Alaska. The first 90 miles of this unprotected coast, from Cross Sound north to the Alsek River, form the west boundary of Glacier Bay National Park.

Inland from this coastal park boundary lies the 30-mile-wide Fairweather Range, cradling huge ice fields. Many of the park's westside glaciers are fed from these vast reservoirs of ice, largest of which is the Brady Icefield. Mount Fairweather, sentinel of the range at 15,320 feet, is higher than any peak in the contiguous United States. In fact, the Fairweather Range is the highest coastal mountain range on the continent. These mountains abut the western shore of Glacier Bay, forming a barrier between the bay and the more severe coastal conditions.

Lithics indicate habitation by humans in this area as early as 10,000 years ago. The Chookenaidi, a sub-group of the Tlingits, had camps in the area when written history of the region was begun by early explorers. Undoubtedly, the tribe had been there for thousands of years, following the glacial ice fronts as they variously advanced and receded in the region. A Chookenaidi oral history recounts the return of ice to Glacier Bay, destroying a village and driving out the residents.

These northern waters support plentiful marine life, a food web that allowed the rich culture of the Tlingits to develop. Many inland native peoples, lacking easy food resources, had little time for creating art as more effort was required for subsistence activities. The elaborate totems and other art forms seen in Southeast Alaska suggest that living here was somewhat easier.

The first sighting of the area by Europeans was in 1741 when the Vitus Bering expedition, accustomed to astounding northern landscapes, passed by and noted the impressive, lofty Fairweather Range. A succession of other sea captains on exploration voyages also passed, leaving wide-eyed descriptions of glacier headwalls in their journals which serve as important benchmarks, locating the position of the ice at the time.

Twelve years after the United States purchased Alaska in 1867, John Muir, well-known naturalist, whose reputation and efforts powered the granting of National Park status to Yosemite, visited Glacier Bay on the first of what were to be four trips. Inspired by what he saw, Muir built a cabin near the glacier that now bears his name, and contributed to the protection effort that was being fostered by the Ecological Society of America and other scientific institutions.

A few, small mining operations, inappropriate in an area of such natural beauty, began in the late years of the 19th Century. Then, in 1924, Calvin Coolidge withdrew about half of the present park area from additional activity, and granted National Monument status and protection in 1925. The monument was increased in size in 1939, and made a National Park in 1980 when half a million acres were added, bringing Glacier Bay National Park to nearly 3.3 million acres. A 57,000-acre preserve was added at the mouth of the Alsek River, at the northern end on the west coast. Full national park protection is administered from the headquarters at Bartlett Cove, just inside the mouth of the bay.

Unlike most national parks, Glacier Bay National Park is actually a marine park, even though the land area within its boundaries greatly exceeds the water area. Here, however, the water is the highway. There is minimal foot-traffic, no trails, and virtually no development in the back-country areas. The only roads are between Bartlett Cove and the nearby town of Gustavus, and only connect those two areas. Vehicles used by residents must arrive by ferry. Visitors travel by boat, or plane.

Geology

How did this immense solitude of waterways and landforms come to be? Glaciation and erosion are responsible for surface contours, while mountain ranges are the result of tectonics. Bedrock origins are varied, complex, and have not been fully studied, especially in the areas more recently uncovered from the ice age.

Earthquakes

Three faults underlie the Glacier Bay area, where tectonic forces from the meeting of the Pacific and Continental plates have caused folding and volcanism. In 1958 a violent, Richter-8 seismic event along the Fairweather fault within the park loosed a major slide at the headwall of Lituya Bay along the outer, Pacific Coast. Huge volumes of rock and ice dropped suddenly into the water, creating a backwash 1,700 feet high that peeled the opposite slope down to bedrock. A huge wave, like a localized, 100'-high tsunami, washed over the entrance to the bay and sank two fishing boats. The backwash scar remains today, souvenir of a quake that caused a 23-foot horizontal displacement along the Fairweather fault. Most events, though, have occurred less abruptly.

Glaciers

Glaciation began here as early as 20 million years ago. Meltback over the last 14,000 years has caused a rebound, or rising of the land surface, as trillions of tons of ice melted. The surface, relieved of tremendous weight, has risen from 300 to 500 feet, and continues to rise today. The Beardslee Island group is rising at a rate of nearly two inches per year.

Prior to 4000 years ago, evidence indicates that the glaciers had withdrawn to near their present location. Mature forests grew along the shores of Glacier Bay then, only to be sheared off at various heights as glaciers again overrode the area. This phenomenon is the source of the interstadial stump forests seen today. Interstadial wood is actually thousands of years old.

Indications exist of glacial balance or thermal equilibrium during long periods of the Little Ice Age beginning about 4,000 years ago. That is, the amount of ice accumulated annually was roughly equalled by the yearly melting, and the glaciers were neither markedly advancing nor receding. Then, in the late 1700s, rapid meltback began. Between 1794 and 1879, 48 miles of Glacier Bay were uncovered. By 1960, Glacier Bay was the same as it is today, give or take a mile here and there. While presently some tidewater glaciers are still receding very slowly, others are again advancing. Glaciologists have determined that short-term weather changes, such as heavier-than-normal snowfall over a period of several years, have no immediate effect on glaciers. Their retreat or advance codes are apparently buried deep within the ice, to be acted upon decades, or centuries, later.

Much evidence of past glaciation is prominent today. Around the south end of Glacier Bay, glaciers at one time scoured peaks to an elevation of 4,200 feet above sea level. Look carefully at the surface contours of the mountains. Glaciated surfaces are smooth and rounded, while peaks extending above the action of glacial ice exhibit sharp, jagged outlines.

There are nearly 200 separate, smaller glaciers in the park in addition to the larger, well-known, tidewater flows. Muir Glacier, once visited frequently by sightseeing ships to observe berg calving, has now retreated and is grounded at the high tide line. Others of note are the Johns Hopkins in an inlet of the same name, and Grand Pacific and Margerie Glaciers in Tarr Inlet, which reach tidewater and present magnificent ice fronts nearly 200 feet high.

Perhaps the most important development at Glacier Bay is the recent large-scale retreat of the tidewater glaciers in the Tarr and Muir inlets. Near these glaciers, the scenery changes every year. Ice may now cover what was a popular viewing spot just a year or so before. At another location, new land area may be uncovered. This short-term change, a continually ongoing feature, plus the compressed-time meltback of the past two centuries, is what makes Glacier Bay such an exciting place.

Plants

Newly uncovered land does not ordinarily remain bare for long. In some areas where glaciers are do-si-doing yearly over the same real estate, or where meandering meltwater streams scour broad outwash surfaces periodically, plants are prevented from securing a root-hold. Such areas remain raw and essentially devoid of plant life as long as these conditions remain.

Most areas newly liberated from perennial ice undergo colonization by plants. First to establish are algae, then mosses and small plant varieties, such as dryas, sedges, grasses, horsetail, and dwarf fireweed. These plants trap wind-borne soil particles in their stands, and provide organic material as they decompose, beginning the process of soil building. Dryas greatly aids the process by fixing nitrogen in the soil.

Next in succession come willows and Sitka alders, growing up through the original colonizers. Alders are important because they build up nitrogen in the soil which other plants need. These larger plants develop into thickets which effectively shade out most smaller competitors. Cottonwood trees grow rapidly, and begin to shade out alders and willows. Sitka spruce seeds, deposited in these thickets by wind, water, or animals, begin to grow slowly in the shade.

Eventually, the young spruce, and later, hemlock trees, reach sunlight, and their growth accelerates. As the trees grow larger, the willows, alders, and cottonwoods are in turn shaded out. Now the two conifers compete with each other during the climax-forest maturation process. In much of the Glacier Bay area, Sitka spruce are the more numerous species at the present time. These are same-age stands, where all the seedlings sprouted at about the same time. It is likely that the climax forest, when eventually stabilized at Glacier Bay, will be predominantly western hemlock.

In some areas of the park, this succession to coniferous forest has happened before, as evidenced by the interstadial stumps previously mentioned. You will see stumps from this ancient forest which grew during opportune times between ice ages, likely more than 4000 years ago. John Muir was especially fascinated by these stumps, and mentioned them at length in his writings. To him they were additional proof of the large-scale advancement and recession of glaciers over time.

There are basically four plant communities in the park. The *Wet Tundra* zone exists at low elevations where level conditions allow standing water. Where drier conditions exist, the *Tundra* moss and plant communities are accomplishing new colonization of bare

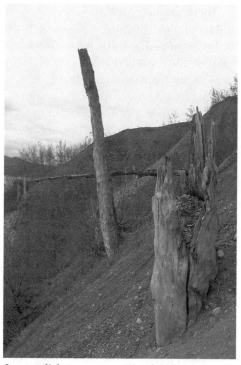

Interstadial stumps near Westdahl Point

areas. At elevations above 2,500 feet, an alpine form of tundra exists that is not succeeded by other communities. *Willow/Alder* communities thrive and expand where they are succeeding the original tundra colonizers. In all but the wettest areas around shorelines and streams, the willow/alder communities are succeeded by *Spruce/Hemlock* forests.

It is easy to observe the more mature forests of spruce and hemlock near the southern end (or mouth) of Glacier Bay, where the land has been uncovered for two centuries. Noticeable, too, is the younger, smaller forest as you move northwards, up-bay, where ice has left more recently. Finally, in the northern inlets, emergence from the ice has been so recent that forests have had little or no time to establish. You will see many vivid examples of varying-age plant communities as you paddle these waters. Glacier Bay continues to be a laboratory for ongoing scientific study of plant succession.

Birds

Over 200 species of birds have been spotted in the park. Of these, only around two dozen are permanent residents. The rest are summer residents, or migrants passing through. The old adage "find the habitat and the food supply, and you will find the bird" holds true here.

Species which you will see often include mew, herring, and glaucous-winged gulls, murres, kittiwakes, puffins, pelagic cormorants, phalaropes, pigeon guillemots, arctic terns, murrelets, and many others. Grebes and loons are plentiful. Shorebirds include black oystercatchers, yellowlegs, sandpipers, plovers, and turnstones, among others. In land environments you will see ptarmigan, ravens, crows, bald eagles, and a host of thrushes, warblers, sparrows, and other species common in the contiguous 48 states.

Because plant communities are older in the southern portions of the bay, certain insect and seed foods are more abundant there. Those birds dependent upon such supplies are naturally more numerous there, also. Look for the greatest variety of birds around meadows, beaches and brushlands, where "edges" between two types of communities provide several different food supplies and cover as well.

Other birds that depend upon the sea for their food supply are most abundant where that marine food web is most easily tapped. Concentrations of small fish attract sea birds. Paddlers commonly see flocks of hundreds of birds, mainly terns and gulls, wheeling and diving into the water, feeding excitedly.

Successful nesting requires food. The rich biodiversity of the bay provides a varied menu, attractive to summer visitors which nest here. Some members of several species which commonly nest farther north, such as the common goldeneye, are lured and short-stopped by food supplies in the area. These birds then nest around the bay. In general, sea birds nest in places not easily accessible to predators, such as on islands or steep cliffs. Birds sense the absence of land predators in the upper fiord areas recently liberated from the ice. In these places, birds establish rookeries as if the mainland shore were an island.

Sea-bird rookeries may be viewed by paddlers without approaching so closely that the birds are disturbed. A pair of compact binoculars is worth bringing, allowing you close views without disrupting wildlife. Do ice worms really exist? Spot a gray-capped rosy finch on a snowfield and observe carefully; you may be able to answer this question for yourself. Be sure to pack a bird guide in your kayak.

Mammals

The large marine mammals of the bay are astonishing and impressive. Humpback whales visit the bay in the summer, arriving from late May through early June after wintering in waters off Mexico and Hawaii. Humpbacks grow to 50 feet in length, and are one species of whale that frequently performs surface displays. It is not uncommon for a humpback to jump partially out of the water several times in succession. If the whale dives steeply, the flukes rise up out of the water, displaying scar and color patterns which scientists use to identify individual whales. Three dozen or more whales may be present in the bay at any one time.

Humpbacks have an interesting feeding method that you may see if you're lucky. After locating a school of small fish, the whale circles the school, emitting a constant stream of bubbles. The bubbles create a circular screen as they rise to the surface, concentrating the fish. The whale then rushes openmouthed through the mass, taking in fish and water. The mouth is closed, water is expelled through baleen plates, and the fish are then swallowed.

While humpbacks appear somewhat tolerant of kayakers, don't take advantage of this and approach too closely. Regulations require that you maintain a distance of one-quarter mile between you and the whales. Occasionally whales swim toward the kayaker and violate that clearance in spite of your good intentions. When this happens, it is both exciting and a little frightening. Though whales have not been known to attack kayakers, their bulk and power can be intimidating when they are right beside your boat.

Orcas, or killer whales, are sometimes seen in the lower portions of bay. The orca is a toothed whale, feeding upon salmon and other fish as well as marine mammal prey such as harbor seals. Minke whales, smallest of the baleen whales, are also present at various times, as are Dall and harbor porpoise. The latter are seen in nearly all portions of Glacier Bay.

Harbor seals and California sea lions may be found in various places in the park. Harbor seals concentrate on ice floes at the heads of inlets in the spring to bear pups. It is almost impossible to kayak any distance in the bay without having the distinctive, rounded head of a harbor seal surface, and look at you with sad, round eyes. Sea lion haul-out spots are mostly on the Pacific Coast of the park.

Undisputed king among land mammals within the region is the brown bear. These coastal forms of grizzly bears range widely over all areas, but are most common in the north and west sections of the park. Black bears inhabit the entire region, but are seldom found in unforested habitats. Both bears are omnivores, making use of a wide range of foods. Black bears can coexist with grizzlies where there are forests for protection. Trees provide a means for the smaller black bears to escape predation from brown bears, which don't climb well.

Preferring brushland and aquatic habitats, moose are common in the park. They are the largest member of the deer family. Their smaller cousins, the blacktail deer, also live in the region but are not plentiful in the park. Mountain goats manage a living on upper slopes, where mosses, lichens and grasses are available. Their long hair is effective insulation, allowing them to remain on exposed mountainsides all winter. They choose slopes where wind and occasional sun help keep snow from accumulating deeper than the animals can dig for food. Mountain goats are most numerous along the eastern shores of the bay. Wolves, like bears, are great travellers; they may be seen anywhere in the park, far from their home range or den sites. Coyotes and red foxes, smaller cousins of the wolf, are found in some areas around Glacier Bay. The foxes are usually seen only at the lower elevations. Both river otters and sea otters are found in Glacier Bay. So are the related mink. Pine martens and wolverines, land cousins of the otters, are sometimes seen, as are weasels. Lynxes may be the sole representative of the cat family. Many different rodents inhabit the area, providing prey for the forest animals.

The key to seeing wildlife is to continually look where you expect it to be. Your quiet passage along the shoreline by kayak is ideal for spotting shy creatures. Search the shore constantly as you paddle; the reward will be many sightings in just a few days. Bring a guidebook to more easily distinguish these animals, as some can be confused with others in their family.

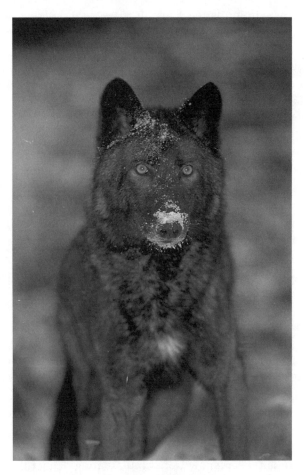

Adult, male gray wolf (black phase)

Chapter 2

Planning Your Trip

To most of us, the purpose of a kayaking trip is enjoyment. This is easy in Glacier Bay, where the aura of this huge fiord system permeates everything. Doing some preliminary planning for your kayak tour will help maximize your enjoyment. There are two basic kinds of trips. One has the physical covering of distance as a major objective. The other is an exploratory trip, where time spent in a small area, getting to know coves, channels, and bays intimately is the main focus. Many trips end up a combination of both. Recognize what is most gratifying to you and then tailor your trip accordingly.

Long-distance paddlers usually see less of the shore—at least at close range. They follow a rigid schedule, where the next campsite must be reached before dark, the tide turns, or the wind comes up. They certainly exhibit physical ability, and competence in expedition logistics. An experienced, trip-hardened paddler could begin at the mouth of Glacier Bay, visit all the inlets, and return to the mouth in 15 days or so. There are those who have done this, and others will do so in the future.

Saving that non-stop, marathon paddling for areas of shoreline that are less interesting, or less sheltered, where passage is best done quickly or on a favorable tide, might be a better idea. Then, as you enter one of Glacier Bay's stunning fiords or bays, you can sit back and breathe the beauty in. For less stress and more fun on a trip, be flexible. But flexibility does not mean carelessness or lack of planning; it means that if conditions indicate that a change of routing or scheduling would be wiser, or more enjoyable, you are willing to make such a change. Plan the ability to change plans.

Planning your trip begins with this book. In addition, other books on general kayaking technique may be helpful to those with less experience; a list of

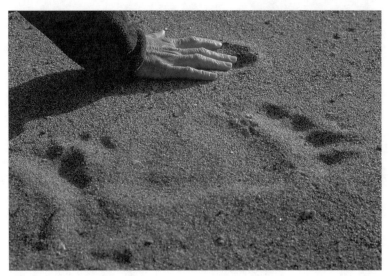

Brown bear track on beach

these is in the Appendix. Gaining an accurate idea of the area and conditions ahead of time is essential when kayak touring. Well-planned trips run smoothly, assuring that most of the surprises are of the pleasant sort. Try to think ahead about all the possibilities and potentials. Contingency planning is good for more than getting you out of an unpleasant situation; it can help you avoid it in the first place. Here are some specific suggestions.

Maps. While no map or chart will prepare you for the beauty and the solitude of Glacier Bay, topographic maps and marine charts are helpful for planning, and absolutely essential for paddling. Marine charts are your means of navigation during the trip. All of Glacier Bay is included on NOAA chart 17318. Topo maps, showing land features and elevations, can also be helpful in recognizing landmarks, and as a guide when you land your boat and go hiking. All the USGS topo maps listed in this book are in the 15-minute series.

Sometimes place names or locations of survey marks which are missing on the marine chart are given on the topo map. This is the case for Glacier Bay maps, and survey marks are used in this text for identifying certain areas. Once you begin paddling, you will easily make the transition from maps to the magnificent scale of the place. Be sure to purchase NOAA chart 17318 and the appropriate topos before you leave on your trip. These maps will not be available at your destination. Map and chart sources are given in the Appendix.

Outfitters. Outfitters who offer commercial kayak trips are a good source of information. Many outfitters are genuinely helpful and will answer specific questions about the areas where they operate, irrespective of whether you book on one of their trips. Such individuals have a keen enthusiasm for the sport of kayaking.

If you are considering a commercial guided trip, match the style of trip offered by the outfitter to your own expectations. Many outfitters do all the work except paddling; with them your paddling days will be short, and you'll spend lots of time in campsites where eating and socializing are main events. Such trips may carry all gear in an accompanying powerboat. Other outfitters offer trips where you share in some of the work, such as cooking or packing, and paddling days may be longer. The trip emphasis may vary greatly between different outfitters, even ones who run trips in the same area.

So if you're leaning toward a commercial trip, research the trip well to make sure you will be comfortable with the style. Ask your prospective outfitter for the names of participants in recent past trips, and phone several of them. If there were any problems with the outfitter, they will likely be mentioned. Participants, most of whom are novices at kayaking, can also tell you if they thought a particular trip was too easy, too hard, etc. Perceptions will vary, of course, but if everyone you contact reports that a certain trip was too hard or too easy for them, consider whether it may be for you also.

Outfitter-planned or Self-planned Trips. Early in your planning decide whether your trip will be an outfitter package, or a self-planned one. Outfitter trips are valuable: if you have never been in a kayak; if you have no companions and would otherwise be paddling solo; or if you just don't want the responsibilities that go along with planning and, even more important, making a trip. Outfitted trips can be very enjoyable. They are an excellent, though not inexpensive, way of sampling the sport of kayaking.

Generally, kayaking with a commercial outfitter is safer than self-planned kayaking in the same waters. One reason is that the outfitter has probably been there before, and has local knowledge that you may not have. Also, few outfitters do trips that truly challenge participants, preferring to accommodate the least capable ones. This tends to keep trips shorter and physical demands less. Just being with a group is a comforting factor when open crossings must be made. Help is quickly available should an unforeseen event occur. Of course outfitted trips have some disadvantages. Your itinerary will be the itinerary of the group. You will leave when the trip leaves, and camp where the outfitter decides to. You will be associating with the other participants for the duration of the trip.

Just because you are not an experienced kayaker does not mean that you should rule out a self-planned trip. Many kayakers in Glacier Bay are on the water for the first time. Just plan your trip within your own capabilities. On self-planned trips, the entire itinerary is your doing. You can alter it along the way to take advantage of those things you most like to see, do, or visit. You can lengthen the trip if you want to, or cut it short. You can decide to paddle

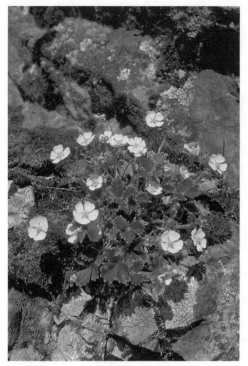
One-flowered cinquefoil, Rendu Inlet

a certain distance on any day, or sit all day among small bergs in a fiord, waiting for the glacier to calve a large one. If there is a favorable tide at midnight, and a moon, you could enjoy an ethereal ghosting down the inlet.

A self-planned trip can be set for any date, to match your schedule and that of your companions. The duration of the trip is up to you, as is the degree of solitude. You decide where your trip begins, and where it ends. If you have had experience on one or two trips, you should be able to plan and execute a kayak trip on your own. If you have never kayaked before, it would be best to plan a modest, unhurried trip. A shorter trip is easier and safer for kayakers while gaining experience. There is less time and distance, over which weather and other conditions can create delays and inconveniences. And the longer the trip, the more any logistical or planning error may have an effect. So let your self-planned trips grow in length and complexity as your experience increases. Balance your abilities to the demands of the trip.

Most trips involve at least two people. They may be either in two, single kayaks, or in a double one. Two people are available to make decisions, and one person to help in the unlikely event that the other is incapacitated. That at least two people kayak together is a very basic safety rule.

Glacier Bay NP. The National Park Service administers Glacier Bay National Park. Knowledgeable rangers can answer your questions, make recommendations, and otherwise help you in trip planning. Free tide tables, regulations, and information brochures are offered. Bear-proof food containers are loaned without charge. Headquarters contacts are listed in the Appendix. Many rangers are kayakers themselves, and their personal experience is of great value. Glacier Bay National Park headquarters contacts are listed in the Appendix.

Time allotment. How long you have to spend is a primary factor in planning any trip. If your time is unlimited, you can organize any kind of trip you desire. Have only one week, or maybe two? Decide what portions of the bay you will be able to see, without hurrying, in that amount of time. A wonderful four or five days can be spent within 6 or 7 miles of the park headquarters. Or, utilizing the day-tour boat for drop-off and pickup service, you can paddle the remote areas and visit glaciers in the same overall amount of time.

Transportation time to and from Glacier Bay is always a factor. It's easy to take the Alaska Marine Highway System ferries from Bellingham, WA to Juneau, and equally easy to take your kayak with you. However, the total ferry time involved from Washington to Glacier Bay and back is six or seven days. Fly to Southeast Alaska and rent a kayak there, and you reduce the transportation time to two days. Then, you can kayak for five days even if you have only one week's vacation. Remember that transportation costs are the same whether your trip is a week or two months in length. Balancing travel logistics to fit your tastes, your must-see areas, and the time available can be an enjoyable part of trip planning. (Transportation suggestions are given in Chapter 3, "Getting There".)

Equipment

Tents. Ideally tents should be no larger than 2-person ones because space to pitch them is often limited. Sturdy, wind-tolerant models that are free-standing, such as the dome types, are best. Free-standing tents are easy to pitch in areas where tent stakes are ineffective, such as soft sand.

Sleeping bags. While extreme temperatures are usually not present in Glacier Bay, moisture often is. Polyester-filled bags are superior to down-filled models because down performs very poorly when it is damp or wet. A compression-type stuff sack greatly reduces the bulk of polyester bags.

Rain gear. Expect drizzle or rain in Glacier Bay. Be sure to include a rain hat with a sufficient brim that water won't drip down inside your collar. If you use a paddling jacket, this garment can double as a rain jacket. A rain shell is a must if you aren't using a paddling jacket. Rain pants offer wind protection ashore, keep you dry when in your boat, and make camp chores more pleasant. Breathable, waterproof rain gear is more comfortable to wear, because of reduced condensation.

Footwear. Wearing knee-high rubber boots while kayaking allows you to get in and out of your boat and still keep your feet dry. The insulated type will help keep your feet warm. Such boots are also comfortable for use around camp and on short hikes. Those desiring a change of footwear for camp use, or contemplating long hikes, may want to take a pair of tennis shoes or hiking boots, as space allows.

Clothing. The most practical fabric for clothing worn next to the skin is polypropelene. Shirts and pants can be of the same material, or of one of the new nylon fabrics which look and feel like cotton. Real cotton is a bad choice for paddling clothing because once wet, it tends to remain wet and has little insulating value. Fleece, or wool, are good choices for shirts and pants. Fleece, however, has little value as a warm outer garment because wind penetrates it so readily. By wearing your rain shell for wind protection over a fleece jacket, you have a layering system that is effective and lightweight.

Stoves. Liquid or propane-fueled stoves are best. There is no wood in many areas of the upper inlets. Make sure to test your stove before leaving home. Some type of wind shield is advisable, as much cooking will be done out in the open. White gas is available in Gustavus and at Glacier Bay Lodge at Bartlett Cove.

Insect protection. Mosquitoes, black flies, and no-see-ums are the flying pests you're most likely to encounter. You will escape these nuisances for the most part while paddling, but ashore in camping areas they can be troublesome. A good deet-based repellent should debug the situation.

Equipment List (may double as packing list)

Boat
- ☐ kayak
- ☐ paddle
- ☐ extra paddle
- ☐ life jacket
- ☐ spray skirt
- ☐ cockpit cover
- ☐ boat-repair kit
- ☐ dry bags
- ☐ bow line
- ☐ additional light line
- ☐ compass
- ☐ chart and maps
- ☐ tide tables
- ☐ paddle float
- ☐ rope self-rescue slings and steps
- ☐ bilge pump
- ☐ sponge
- ☐ water canteen

Safety
- ☐ wet suit or dry suit
- ☐ flares
- ☐ signal mirror
- ☐ weather radio
- ☐ barometer or altimeter

☐ matches or lighter (in separate, waterproof container)*
☐ hand-held transceiver (Optional)**

* Stove fuel, or the lighted stove itself, are excellent emergency firestarters.
** Because ranger patrols are infrequent and the bay is so large, securing aid in emergencies could be difficult. A small VHF transceiver allows contact with boats travelling the main routes in the bay.

Camping
☐ tent with fly, stakes & wind guys, & extra nylon cord
☐ sleeping bag & pad
☐ stove
☐ fuel for stove
☐ matches & lighter kept with stove
☐ cooking pot
☐ bowl
☐ spoon
☐ cup
☐ water filter or treatment tablets
☐ water bags or containers for 2-day supply

Food
Food is highly personal. We carry:

Breakfast
　instant oatmeal
　brown sugar
　Tang
　powdered hot chocolate

Lunches and snacks
　trail mix with lots of nuts, dried fruit
　shelled sunflower seeds
　dried apricots
　dried pineapple slices
　granola bars or energy bars

Dinners
　pre-cooked freeze-dried dinners
　powdered hot chocolate

We do not like to spend time cooking when on kayaking trips, so the above menu works well for us, while providing a sufficiently balanced diet with enough calories to keep going for long periods. One additional benefit to pre-cooked, freeze-dried food is that there is no cooking odor to attract bears.

There are as many variations in food preferences as there are people, so work out your own. Remember that even though a kayak offers generous cargo space, weight and bulk are still considerations. Add to this the present requirement that all food carried by paddlers within the park *must* be carried in bear canisters, and you have all the more reason to go light and compact.

Clothing List
- [ ] underwear (polyester such as Capilene)
- [ ] long johns, tops & bottoms (polyester such as Capilene)
- [ ] socks (wool or poly)
- [ ] shirt (poly or nylon)
- [ ] pants (poly or nylon)
- [ ] pile jacket
- [ ] paddling jacket or rain jacket
- [ ] gloves or pogies (hand protection attached to paddle shaft)
- [ ] hat with brim (for shade and rain drip)
- [ ] rubber boots
- [ ] hiking boots

Personal
- [ ] prescription medications
- [ ] prescription glasses with strap
- [ ] sun glasses with strap
- [ ] first-aid kit
- [ ] wilderness medicine book
- [ ] sun screen (15 and above)
- [ ] insect repellent
- [ ] personal toiletry items
- [ ] camera & film
- [ ] mini binoculars
- [ ] entertainment items (books, cards)

Volumes can be written about what items to take and not to take. The above equipment list is very basic, with most items either used daily, or necessary for reasonable safety. Beyond these lists, equipment is strictly individual preference. A camera and film, for example, are clearly discretionary items, but who would go without them? A wilderness medical guide will probably never be utilized, but will you leave it home? What will you do all day if storms keep you tent-bound? Books are heavy and bulky. Do you really need binoculars?

Apply this test to each equipment item: Can you get along without it? Or, for safety items: Is deleting this item an unacceptable risk? Obviously, you can't get along without your paddle; you won't leave your life jacket behind. Final equipment lists, though, always include some discretionary trade-offs of extra bulk and weight being tolerated because the item is desired.

Chapter 3

Kayaking In Glacier Bay

When To Go

What is the best time to kayak Glacier Bay? There may be little choice of dates for you because of set vacations or other schedules. Or you may be fortunate to have greater flexibility, and can plan a trip during any portion of "the paddling season." The Park Service opens its back-country office a few days after the first of May. During May and June there is the greatest chance of extended periods of clear weather in Glacier Bay. Prior to May, weather conditions may be harsher than you wish to experience, with snow flurries possible, and low temperatures. Around the end of June, periods of precipitation are more likely, increasing in frequency on through the summer. September offers a good chance of periodic sunshine, often better than in midsummer. October at this latitude means that winter has begun, with occasional snow likely, and generally cold temperatures.

The cruise ship season begins in April and runs through mid-October. Since only two large ships are allowed in Glacier Bay each day, the only way cruise lines can increase the number of paying passengers is to extend the season. But cruise-ship passengers do not brave the elements like kayakers do; you can view through glass on a ship, remaining warm and snug in spite of the weather. Those who go on deck can go back inside at any time. Because inclement weather is tolerable—even exciting—for passengers, the cruise ship industry has expanded into the shoulder seasons.

Weather

Most of the region's storms are spawned in the Gulf of Alaska. The Gulf of Alaska and the Aleutian Island chain lie in a region where warm southwesterly, Pacific currents meet colder air and water from the Bering Sea. The clash produces unstable air, causing precipitation with little warning. Such a disturbance revolves counterclockwise while it is swept generally eastward by northern hemispheric winds. Reaching the Alaska coast, it moves ashore and provides more precipitation. Before reaching Glacier Bay, a storm hits the Fairweather Range, which forces the moisture-laden air upward. The resultant cooling condenses the moisture, which falls as snow on the mountains. This snow augments the ice fields feeding the glaciers.

Some moisture survives lifting by the mountains to fall as precipitation in the rain shadow east of the Fairweathers. At Bartlett Cove near the mouth of Glacier Bay, 30 miles east, precipitation averages 75 inches annually, 40 percent less than farther west. Since Bartlett Cove is not fully protected by high ridges to the west as are the northern portions of the bay, expect precipitation at the northern end of Glacier Bay to be lighter, and of shorter duration.

Fog is common in Icy Strait at the mouth of the bay. The marine environment guarantees moisture, and there is no shortage of cold air from ice fields and glaciers. When the moisture in the air is cooled to the point of condensing, fog can occur. Sometimes the fog rolls in; at other times the gray mist seemingly materializes, even when just a short time before it was clear. As you move north up Glacier Bay, the likelihood of fog decreases. Around the upper inlets, you can often enjoy clear skies while to the south, fog, low clouds or drizzle dampen the area.

Wind

Because much of the water in Glacier Bay is sheltered, a kayaker can usually avoid very rough water. Yet, in a body of water over 60 miles long and up to 10 miles wide, wind must be considered. Understanding and using the wind patterns likely to be encountered on your trip will maximize your enjoyment by minimizing unnecessary effort.

The long, narrow configuration of the various inlets might indicate that winds, unless they are blowing parallel to the inlet, don't have a long sweep in which to build up waves. However, winds have a tendency to follow the terrain, and when this happens, sizable wind waves can result. Luckily there are many coves and smaller inlets along Glacier Bay that provide calm water. Many kayakers plan their entire trip around these spots, or at least plan to camp at them. Inlets or bays which lie at an angle to the prevailing winds generally provide calm waters. The trip descriptions in this book frequently mention these protected areas.

To locate calm areas or landing spots, which are sheltered from the wind, look for lees. Lees are that side of any mountain, shoreline, island, or rock, which is protected from the wind. Using a small island as an example, when the wind is blowing from the north, the lee of the island is on the south side. Similarly, when the wind is blowing parallel to a shoreline, any small cove or point which protects a segment of the shoreline running at an angle to the main shore will provide a lee.

In some cases, a sheltering point may be so small that it is not shown on your chart. Usually, though, shoreline contours will show indications of possible spots to duck into if things get rough. Even barriers as unlikely as a bed of kelp can provide protection from waves caused by wind, even though the wind itself passes on unimpeded. Experienced kayakers always look ahead for such places, and keep them in mind should conditions change.

Winds associated with weather fronts tend to come from the southwest in Glacier Bay. Prevailing winds during periods of clear weather are usually from the north, blowing down-bay. Even when overall wind patterns are from the prevailing direction, winds at the water's surface often follow along the larger inlets, channeled by the steep shorelines. This can result in breezes in these inlets that blow at right angles to the prevailing direction.

Gravity winds, also called glacial winds, are formed when air is cooled by contact with glaciers or ice fields. This cold air is at first stationary over the ice. But cold air is heavier than warmer air, and eventually the cold mass flows down the glacier and out into the inlet or bay. Gravity winds can form in the least expected location with little notice any time of day or night, and are sometimes quite strong. Glacial winds usually blow parallel to the inlet in which they are encountered.

When To Paddle

Don't launch if the wind is blowing strong enough to make you uneasy. Stay within your comfort zone. Kayakers sometimes spend a day or two in camp, waiting for favorable conditions. That is part of the adventure, and is far preferable to feeling that you *must* launch and make progress, risking conditions that tax your capabilities. Fortunately, many factors in Glacier Bay work in favor of the kayaker.

As in most areas, Glacier Bay winds are more likely to arise in the afternoon, when surface warming occurs. So calmer mornings are the preferred paddling times. In many instances, relative calm prevails all day, but mornings are the more reliable time to expect good, smooth paddling conditions. Paddle quite close to shore when conditions are uncertain. Doing this makes it easy to get ashore quickly. If you are a mile from shore and conditions deteriorate, it will take you at least 20 minutes to reach sheltering landforms. Learn to "quarter" large waves. Several books on kayaking technique offer valuable advice to beginners on basic boat handling and seamanship. Books on kayaking technique are listed in the Appendix.

Safety In Cold Water

Because Glacier Bay waters are very cold, especially in the upper inlets, paddling here presents a hazard. An unprotected paddler in the water can become incapacitated in a very short time. The only way to stop the rapid heat loss from immersion is to end the contact with cold water.

While the likelihood of capsizing is slight for careful paddlers, having an emergency plan is wise. Many experienced kayakers recommend wearing wet or dry suits which insulate the body. Such suits also provide warmth while paddling in inclement weather by shedding rain, spray, and stopping wind. Absolutely essential is the ability to right your boat, and climb back in. Many self-rescue techniques are taught at kayak schools and clubs. Learn a practical method and practice until you master it. The Park Service states that the best safety strategy for paddlers in very cold water is to keep their boats upright. Apparently that advice works; large numbers of kayakers ply Glacier Bay waters each season without incident.

Safety Around Ice

You will paddle among icebergs if you visit the upper portions of Muir Inlet or the upper, west arm of Glacier Bay. If you work your way close to a calving glacier, you will likely be surrounded by icebergs. The only way to approach a tidewater glacier is to weave through ice pack and bergs, following lanes of open water. Bergs are heavy and unyielding; running into one can damage your kayak.

Dangerous situations can occur when bergs begin to close ranks, and the open lanes of water are restricted or disappear. You can be lured deep inside ice packs when the ebb tide separates the bergs and spreads them out along the fiord. But when flood tide begins, the bergs move together again, and open lanes may close. Do not remain in an ice pack when a flood tide is compressing it. Individual bergs present unseen dangers. Since the melting process underwater is more rapid than above, bergs eventually become unstable and turn or roll over. If you are too close when the berg shifts, any underwater shelf or projection on the berg can flip your boat. Just the wave disturbance alone could capsize you.

Just as bergs calve from the glacier face above water, the underwater melting process occasionally calves bergs from the glacier's underwater face. Being buoyant and hydrodynamically irregular, such bergs can shoot to the surface unexpectedly, and at considerable distance from the glacier.

Tides And Currents

Unlike areas where island groups and intersecting straits create confusing patterns of tidal currents, current directions in Glacier Bay are generally very

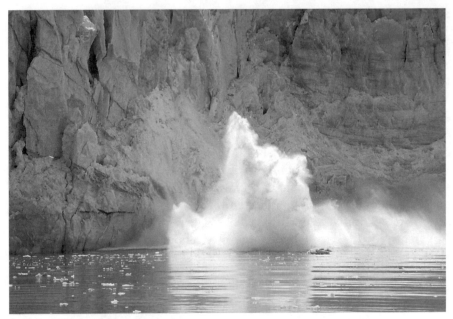

Lamplugh Glacier calves

clear. When the tide is flooding, currents will run north, toward the heads of bays and inlets. On the ebb tide, currents run to the south. Where the inlets do not lie north and south, just remember that the ebb tide flows toward the mouth of the bay, and the flood toward the head of the inlet. Scidmore Bay and Charpentier Inlet, branching as a T off Hugh Miller Inlet, have currents that run toward the stem of the T on ebb, and from the stem toward the heads of the bays on flood tide.

Current direction around islands is a different matter, especially if there are two or more islands in close proximity. Tidal flows can "feed" the area behind the island from either side. What actually does happen is controlled by channel depth, current mass and velocity, as well as underwater topography.

There are many ways to determine current direction and speed. Simply stop paddling for a time, and estimate drift direction and speed by observing your movement in relation to the shoreline, or nearby rocks. The common seaweed kelp, which grows anchored to the bottom and reaches long fronds to the surface, makes an excellent current indicator. The slightest flow will cause the surface portion of the plant to point along the direction the current is moving.

In any place where a large water body is constricted like the lagoon at McBride Glacier, Scidmore Bay, or other bays with narrow entrances, as well as Sitakaday Narrows, current velocity increases over that of surrounding areas. The only way for the water volume to pass through the narrows in a given amount of time is to increase velocity. Such areas should be avoided by kayakers during times of strong currents. Some lagoon areas off the smaller bays develop tidal rapids on ebb tides, at least one of which is roaring white-water and not possible to negotiate.

As a flood tide changes to ebb tide, and as ebb changes to flood, there is a period known as slack water. While it may be almost imperceptible, remember that for some time before slack water, and some time after, there is a period of relative still water when paddling even the most constricted spot is possible. If you start paddling 30 minutes before slack water, and paddle 30 minutes after the tide change, you will travel around 3 miles. Usually this is far enough to pass safely through strong current areas. In this example, you will paddle half the time against a weak current, and receive a boost for half the time from an equally weak current. Slack water periods occur approximately every six hours.

The strongest current period is from one hour after slack water, until one hour before the next slack water at tide change. Remember that you paddle around 3 miles per hour. It makes little sense to try to paddle against a 3 miles per hour current, or even one going 2 miles per hour. Rather, plan your paddle taking wind and current into consideration. Current speed in Glacier Bay varies greatly from less than one-half knot near the heads of inlets and in the broad sections of the bay, to more than 6 knots near the entrance to the bay and in various constricted areas.

Currents become dangerous when they are sufficiently strong to create whirlpools and large boils. Either of these can upset an unwary kayaker. In some locations, tiderips, which are like stationary waves, are present. Rips pose a real threat to paddlers. Luckily, these types of hazards can be predicted, and are quite visible when present.

Be sure to bring a tide table. Glacier Bay tides at the mouth average 15 minutes later than times listed for Juneau. Near the north end of the bay, tides occur about 30 minutes after the Juneau times listed in the tables.

Eddies

Points projecting out from shore often create areas where currents, immediately downstream from the point and very close to shore, are flowing in the opposite direction from the flow in the main channel. These helpful currents are known as back eddies. This phenomenon can extend hundreds of yards down from the point, providing a welcome boost if you have to make progress against the main current.

Small islands also provide some diminishing of currents close to their downstream shores. Tidal currents moving across shallow areas flow more slowly than in mid-channel, where obstructions are absent and the greatest volume of water moves. But if the only course available to the current flow is over a shallow area, the current moves much faster than if the water was deep. Since kayakers make progress by muscle power, such phenomenon are quickly learned, and put into immediate practice.

Launching And Landing

Most landing and launching places in the inlets and coves of Glacier Bay are in calm water. No special surf landing skills are required, such as those necessary in exposed coastal kayaking. Many beaches are of small gravel or shingle, easy to land upon and forgiving to kayak bottoms. There are mud shorelines in places, and some locations where extensive mud flats are exposed at low water. Generally, it is not difficult to recognize these areas and avoid them in favor of gravel beaches. Trip descriptions in this book mention the type of beach at many campsites. There is no shortage of good landing beaches. They are plentiful along all shores except where cliffs and steep slopes drop abruptly into the water. Many of these limited landing areas are described in the trip narratives.

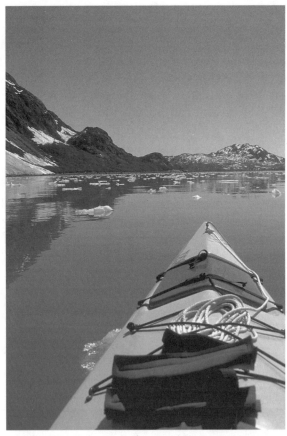

If you make a rest stop, or longer for lunch, make sure you keep an eye on the tide. *Always* tie your bow line to something solid before you walk away from the boat. A rising tide can float your kayak in a matter of minutes, and a wind gust or slight current could take it out of reach seconds later. Near the head of

Paddling Tarr Inlet on a calm morning

inlets with calving ice, unexpected swells of 2 or 3 feet are possible, raising havoc with improperly beached boats. If feasible, move your kayak to a secure spot several feet above the water in these areas, and tie the bow line securely.

Non-Motorized Areas

Several motorless areas have been established in Glacier Bay during various seasons to enhance the wilderness experience of paddlers. In these areas you are free from anglers and sightseers in motorized vessels, as well as smaller "eco-tour" cruise ships. You may still see a cruise ship miles away, or a smaller day-tour boat near the edge of the closed area. Non-motorized restrictions change as closures are ordered by the Park Service for certain areas for specified time periods. At this writing, motorless areas during various times in the paddling season include: the Beardslee Islands, Adams Inlet, Wachusett Inlet, Muir Inlet, Rendu Inlet, and the Hugh Miller-Scidmore complex.

Permits

You need a back-country permit from the Park Service before beginning your kayak trip. Permits are routinely issued free of charge at the back-country office near the dock at Bartlett Cove. Be sure to check with the Park Service during the planning stages of your trip. Quotas may be filled, or new regulations be in place which you need to know about.

Coinciding with receiving your permit, you get a kayaker orientation. The purpose is to inform you of park regulations, make sure you know about closures in effect, and generally give you the data necessary to comply with regulations and safely enjoy your trip in the park. Bear canisters are provided at this time. The back-country office at Bartlett Cove is open around the first week in May, from 7:00 A.M. to 9:00 P.M. daily, until mid-September. Contact information for Glacier Bay National Park is given in the Appendix.

Getting There

You cannot drive to Juneau, Alaska, much less to Bartlett Cove. Access is by boat or air. The Alaska Marine Highway System ferries sail weekly from Bellingham, Washington, to Juneau, Alaska. Travel time is around two and one-half days, one way. Kayaks are carried aboard the ferries for a modest fee in addition to the regular passenger fare. From Juneau, a passenger-carrying catamaran runs daily to Gustavus, and can accommodate kayaks. This boat docks at Gustavus, ten miles by road from Bartlett Cove. A taxi service in Gustavus has a van with top racks which can transport kayaks to the launching site.

Alaska Marine Highway System ferries also depart from Prince Rupert, on the British Columbia coast 800 highway miles northwest of Bellingham. Fare from Prince Rupert to Juneau is considerably less than from Bellingham.

Using the Alaska ferries is the only inexpensive and practical way of transporting a rigid kayak to Glacier Bay.

If you have a collapsible kayak, which packs into one or two large bags, you can consider flying to Glacier Bay, and take your collapsible along. Flying is quick, and there are good schedules from the Seattle area to Juneau. It may be necessary to pay extra baggage charges for your boat. From Juneau, you have a choice of taking the daily ferry to Gustavus, or flying there.

Another possibility is to rent a kayak from the concessionaire at Bartlett Cove or one of the private outfitters in Gustavus. With a boat reserved at your put-in point, you can either journey to the park by ferry or by air. Several outfitting companies operate kayaking trips in Glacier Bay. These are guided trips, where all gear is supplied except your personal items. All you need to do is to show up. Contact information for the Alaska State Marine Highway System, Juneau-to-Gustavus ferry, airlines, kayak-rental sources, and outfitters are given in Appendix 1.

Drop-Off Trip Options

From Bartlett Cove, a tour boat operated by Glacier Bay Lodge makes a daily round trip to the head of Tarr Inlet at the north end of Glacier Bay. Arrangements can be made to take kayaks and paddlers to one of three drop-off points in the bay. This valuable service makes it possible for kayakers on limited schedules to visit even the most remote areas of the park.

For instance, you can schedule a drop-off near the entrance to Muir Inlet, paddle that winding wilderness for a week, then be picked up again where you were let off. Or, you can arrange a food drop to allow a more lengthy paddle without being overburdened with supplies. Many different trip options are possible utilizing the drop-of service. Currently, drop-off points are at Mt. Wright near the entrance to Muir Inlet, Glacier Bay near the north Scidmore Bay tidal channel, and Geikie Inlet on the west shore. Contact information for the drop-off service is given in Appendix 1.

Chapter 4

Camping In Glacier Bay

Shoreline Camping and Site Selection

In most areas of the bay, campsites are not difficult to find. Encroaching alders often limit otherwise excellent camping beaches, but many areas are clear, offering sufficient room for a small tent either on fine gravel or grass. When given a choice, avoid plant areas and choose to camp on the gravel where the disturbance you make will have minimum impact. Finding a tent site that is reasonably level *and* above any possible high water is the goal. Since fresh water is available from so many sources and easily carried, camping by water is not a necessity.

In evaluating a tent site, several criteria should be considered. First, the site needs to be above any high water. Second, the area should not be flooded or puddled if it rains. Third, the area should be level, or only as sloping as you are willing to tolerate. Fourth, but not necessarily last, the site should not be on a bear trail or in a high use area for bears. Other considerations are shelter from wind, and proximity to fresh water.

Look for tent sites where streams have formed outwash fans along the shore. Often these fans are newly formed, and vegetation is limited. Beaches in such places are frequently gravel. Look along shores where gravel beaches are evident. Islands often offer good camp sites, in coves and near each end along the direction of glacier movement. Be sure to check your chart for extensive mud flats near the campsite, to avoid marooning yourself. Another good place to find tent sites is on points jutting out from the mainland. Points often mean a protected landing beach is present.

Coves, regardless of size, often provide snug camping sites. Protection is usually good, unless the wind blows directly into the cove. Beaches and coves often go hand in hand. You may be surprised at the amount of shelter offered by even the tiniest cove along a rocky shore. A landing beach is a necessity, as is a tent site that is well above the high-water mark. Don't get caught in a tiny cove as the tide is inching around your tent and your retreat is cut off by a vertical rock face.

Determine the high-water mark by observing any flotsam such as driftwood or seaweed on the beach. If you can identify the height of the most recent, previous high tide, you can check in the tide tables for a relationship to the next high tide. Be sure to allow a safety margin, for tide tables have been in error, and observations are not always foolproof. Remember that green rye grass on the upper portion of the beach does not mean that the area is above the highest tide level. Check your tide table for those periodic, unusually high tides.

In some locations, you will find old, wave-formed gravel shelves that are ideal for camping. These may be many feet above the present high-water line. Thank the fact that the land is rising rapidly for any such ideal spot. Many of these shelves are now covered with alder to varying degrees. They make

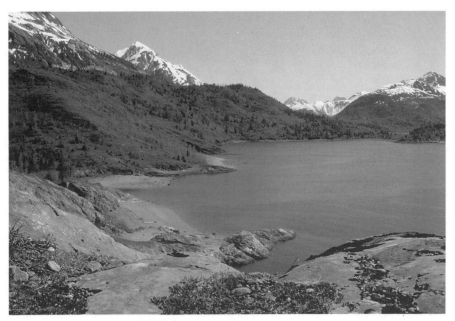

Glacier Bay campsite near Tidal Inlet

ideal, sheltered camps when there is sufficient room between alders for your tent, but the view is hampered or nonexistent, and you can't see approaching bears.

If you camp close to calving glaciers, take into account the possibility of 2-3' surge waves. Remember to tie up your boat. You can continue your trip with a wet tent and soggy gear, but lose your boat, and you're in for an embarrassing wait.

Since some of the better tent sites are in exposed locations, your tent should be capable of withstanding moderate to strong winds. Attaching extra guy lines to loops or fasteners on the fly will improve the strength of most tents. Most campsites, being on fine gravel or sand, will offer little purchase for tent stakes. Be sure to tie a 4'-long piece of stout nylon cord onto each stake loop on your tent. If your fly has storm guys, make sure these are extra long. This will allow you to tie to rocks for use as anchors in place of stakes. If it gets really windy, add more rocks. It is good etiquette to scatter these rocks when you leave to eliminate traces of your use.

A small, light-weight tarp is handy in case of extended rains. Use it as a shelter to cook under. (In no circumstances should you cook in your tent. The resulting food odors are bad news in bear country.) The tarp can also be used to cover the pile of gear that came out of your boat, protecting it from dew or precipitation.

Water

There is an abundance of fresh water in Glacier Bay. Melt streams from annual snows and perennial streams separate from glaciers are the best bet for water which does not have silt, or glacial flour in it. These streams are found in all areas of the bay. Late in the year, after lower elevation snows have melted, such flows are less numerous. Still, it is a rare section of shoreline that does not have usable water every mile or two. Be sure to treat or filter your drinking water, even if it appears clear. Cooking water need not be treated if it is boiled during the cooking process. Use of a storage container, such as a water bag, allows you to carry sufficient water for overnight camping.

The larger streams, especially glacial melt streams, carry a great deal of silt and glacial flour. If you must use water from a silted stream, allow it to stand long enough for most of the suspended material to settle and then pour off the clear water before filtering or chemically treating it.

Sanitation

Dispose of body waste as low as possible within the intertidal zone. Utilize a rocky area, not the same smooth beach used for landing. Tidal action will flush your waste, and its decomposition is assured. Burn all excess toilet paper unfolding as much of it as possible before lighting.

Fires

Wood fires, although they awaken some primal instincts in all of us, are not environmentally sound in the wilderness. Small stoves are recommended instead. While wood fires are not prohibited by the Park Service, the evidence of campfires is unsightly. Many areas in Glacier Bay have a very limited wood supply because trees have not had time to become established. Decaying wood provides nutrients that are needed in the soil. If you must have a wood fire, build it below the high-water mark. That way, the tide will sweep all signs of your fire away within a short time.

Burning interstadial wood is prohibited. Such wood has scientific value in the field of dendrochronology because of its great age. Interstadial wood is found in chunks as driftwood, in the form of logs, and as stumps still rooted at the site of inter-ice-age forests.

Bears And Bear Closures

Both brown bears and black bears are abundant in the park. Both are very intelligent animals that learn quickly. One incident is enough to imprint an event on the memory of a bear. Easily habituated then, bears can be a problem if they come to view humans as deliverers of food. It is extremely important that bears not be afforded the opportunity to secure food from humans. Bears that form this habit are dangerous, as they loose their natural fear of humans. Usually, once a bear becomes a "problem," it must be destroyed.

Intertidal areas provide natural food for both bear species. The occasional dead fish, sea bird or crustacean that washes ashore is easy pickings for bears, and they know it. Bears feed heavily on barnacles and mussels in the intertidal zone at certain times of the year. Consequently, some animals establish routes to patrol along shore, especially in estuaries and coves. Easily available food supplies always concentrate bears. This happens seasonally when salmon run up streams and rivers flowing into the bay. Spawning salmon usually attract lots of bears.

When bear concentrations reach a certain point, or when reports of bear activity indicate that caution be exercised, the Park Service will initiate a bear closure of the area. This means it is closed to people camping in the area. You can go ashore in a bear closure area, but you cannot camp there overnight.

In 1997 there was a bear closure in effect for the east shore of Glacier Bay, from Wolf Creek north almost to Muir Point. Camping was allowed on Sturgess and Leland Islands, making it possible to paddle from Bartlett Cove to Muir Inlet without facing a long paddle between camps. Very numerous black bears in the area were the reason for this closure. A bear closure was also in effect on the west side of Tarr Inlet from Margerie Glacier to Jaw Point in Johns Hopkins Inlet. This closure was a result of brown bear activity.

The Park Service requires use of bear canisters for food transport and storage. Canisters are smooth cylinders with flush ends, made of strong plastic or metal. Because they are large enough that a bear cannot get its teeth around them, and because the surface is slippery and offers no tooth or claw hold, bears cannot open the canisters. People can, using a coin or slot screwdriver.

The proper way to use storage canisters is to remove only that food which you will cook and eat immediately, and place the remainder back into the canister and close it. At night, do not store the canister in your tent, and don't leave it in your kayak. If there are no trees to hang the canister, leave it out in the open a good distance from your tent. Bear canisters of various sizes are provided by the park service. Select from 8x12, 8x18, 10x14 and 10x18 inch sizes. The 8x18" size will hold carefully selected food for two people for a week, on average.

Walking, hiking, or just being on shore creates the chance of a bear encounter. Most bears shy away from humans if they are given an opportunity to do so. But they don't like surprises. When walking on land in areas where alder, forest, or terrain limits visibility, be sure to announce your presence by making noise. Forget bear bells, or rocks in a tin can. Use your voice, with good volume, a couple of times each minute that you are in any area

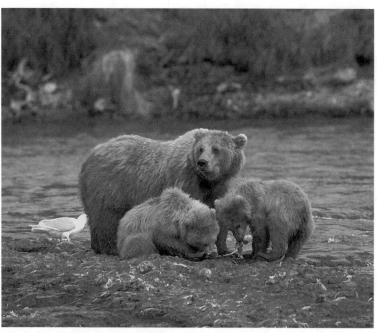

Alaska brown bear with cubs eating salmon catch

where visibility is limited. Clapping your hands a few times each minute while you are moving through thick cover is effective in letting bears know you are there.

Few people realize how well bears can detect odors. Smell is the most important sense the animals utilize in finding food. To avoid attracting bears to food scents, keep a clean camp. Improper food storage, or even tiny bits of food spilled on the ground may attract bears. Candy-bar wrappers carelessly stuffed in a jacket pocket are enough to attract bears to the garment. The use of strongly scented cosmetics should be avoided. Make sure the sunscreen lotion you take is not scented. The same goes for soaps, or any substance that will transfer scent that might be mistaken for food to your body or clothes. Pamphlets with suggestions for minimizing chances of bear encounters are available from the Park Service.

Fishing

Sport fishing is allowed in the Glacier Bay National Park, as well as some commercial fishing. The latter is presently undergoing an evaluation of its impact on park ecosystems. Because State of Alaska regulations apply, you will need a fishing license, which is available in Gustavus and at Bartlett Cove if you haven't purchased one on your way to the park. Salmon, steelhead, and trout are the salmonids in the bay. Of course halibut are common, as are other bottom fish.

If you decide to fish, it will probably be to vary your diet or extend your food supply, but it may be just for sport. Use extreme care around camp when cleaning and cooking fish. All cleaning and cooking should be done in the intertidal zone. If you are careless and leave fish or scraps, cooked or uncooked, you are likely to receive a visit from a bear. Be sure to thoroughly wash any dishes or utensils used for fish. Do this in tidewater, so the odor will be carried away. Don't wipe your hands on your clothing. Don't take tainted clothing into your tent at night.

How To Use This Book

Maps. NOAA chart 17318 is the one to use for navigation in Glacier Bay. **The maps in this book are intended for familiarization only, and not for navigation purposes.** Trip descriptions include survey marks found only on USGS topographic maps, in the 15-minute series. Be sure you have the proper maps before you go.

Mileage. Three mileage estimates are used in the trip descriptions. The first is given at the beginning of each trip chapter, as the length of the trip. The second group of mileage figures are used in the narrative as the distance between places. A third group of mileage figures are in parenthesis, and represent the distance paddled since the beginning of the trip.

Distance figures between places are usually rounded to the nearest one-half (0.5) mile. If the distance is less than that, it may be stated in tenths of a mile. The cumulative effect of variation in the distance-between-places mileage is that the actual trip length may vary somewhat. Also, the amount of exploration and number of detours, even tiny ones, will affect the distance that you actually paddle on the trip.

Time. Time, given as the number of days, is an estimate only. You may find a multitude of things you want to explore in, say, Adams Inlet, and to accomplish that you might spend a week there. Another paddler might spend two days in Adams Inlet and, satisfied, be ready to move on. Use the number of days as a rough guide, but if you spend less time than the minimum suggested, you might be missing something.

Rating. A trip is rated "Easy" if there are no likely physical conditions which require more than basic, beginner kayaking skills. A "Moderate" rating is applied if kayaking conditions are sometimes, or are usually, difficult enough that some experience with rough water and wind is advisable. "Difficult" ratings denote trips where open crossings are necessary, or long sections of unprotected shorelines must be paddled. The "Difficult" rating indicates the likelihood of rough conditions is high, and you must have experience with such conditions in order to paddle there safely.

Campsites. Throughout the trip chapters reference is made to proven and possible campsites. Many of these locations have been used by the author and by other kayakers. Other spots have been scouted, and found to be feasible for camping. Rating campsites is difficult. For some kayakers, a view is the decisive feature in making a choice. Others must have a site that is beside or near a stream. A protected site is desirable in windy weather. It is rare when any one spot fulfills all these requirements. For this reason, little attempt has been made to qualify camping sites. In locations where landing spots are scarce, and flat spots even less numerous, *any* place where a tent can be pitched safely above high water qualifies as a good camp. If you are dissatisfied with the site you find at one location, you can paddle on to the next possible locale and search there. Scarcity of good campsites is a primary reason for identifying a site early in the day, in case you need to investigate several before finding a spot you consider adequate.

Trip Descriptions. There are 12 trips described in the following chapters. Cumulatively, they represent over 300 miles of paddling along the shorelines of Glacier Bay. These trips, if done in order, will basically take you on a counterclockwise circumnavigation of Glacier Bay including all of its inlets and coves. Most paddlers will not do all the trips consecutively. To do so would require from three to six weeks. Few people have that kind of free time. Thanks to the fine drop-off service provided by Glacier Bay Lodge, you can paddle to the most remote spot in the bay in a matter of two or three days.

This enables you to select a single trip, or a combination of two or more, depending upon the amount of time you have available. A few trips are located some distance from the drop-off points, and to reach the starting point of these trips, all or a portion of the previous trip must be paddled. When this is the case it is noted at the beginning of the trip description. Data in this book has been gathered from paddling notes of the author while kayaking, suggestions from park personnel and other kayakers, and research.

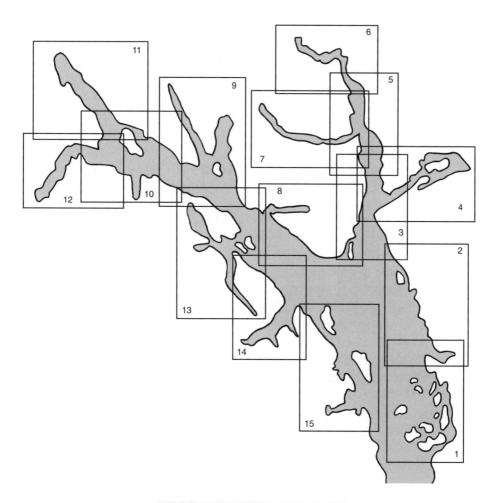

MAPS IN THIS BOOK

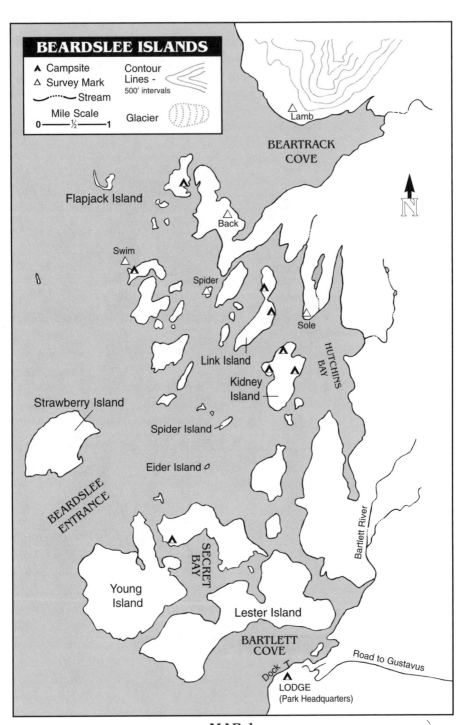

MAP 1

Chapter 5

 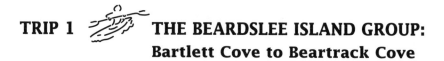 **THE BEARDSLEE ISLAND GROUP:**
Bartlett Cove to Beartrack Cove

Trip Details

Distance:	29 miles RT from Bartlett Cove (33 miles RT with Beartrack Cove option) 12 miles one way from Bartlett Cove to Beartrack Cove
Time:	2-7 days
Rating:	Easy
Maps:	NOAA Chart 17318; USGS Topos: Juneau (B-6) & (C-6)

Summary and Highlights

The protected, narrow waterways, wooded islands, and good camping found among the Beardslee Islands makes this the ideal destination for a very relaxing paddle. The lack of harsh conditions appeals to first-time kayakers. The sea and shore birds, seals, land mammals, and views of the Fairweather Range make the Beardslee Islands a memorable destination. The Beardslee Island waters are classified as non-motorized from May 15 through September 15. In addition, certain landing and approach restrictions apply to specific areas to avoid disturbance to wildlife. Check the current regulations at the park headquarters before setting out from Bartlett Cove. The major hazard on this trip is the cold water. Survival time in water colder than 45° Fahrenheit is very short.

Area Features, Background, and Tips

The Beardslee Island group is made up of over three dozen islands at high tide, and many more at low water when rocks and shoals are exposed. The

islands are located immediately north of Bartlett Cove. Some scientists theo-
rize that the Beardslees were deposited as the last glacier melted northward,
uncovering the bay in the 1700s.

The greatest elevation of any island in the Beardslee group is just over 200
feet, found on a 2-mile-long, unnamed island northeast of Young Island. Most
islands are quite low, and gentle in slope. The present 2"-annual uplift means
that not only are the islands increasing in elevation and new islands appear-
ing, but the water around them is decreasing in depth. Channels that were
passable just a few years ago are not usable today.

Of the many rocks and shoal areas exposed at low tide, most but not all are
shown on the marine chart. Running onto a rock could produce scratches, or
a cracked hull. Kayakers can avoid such problems in the Beardslees both by
checking the chart carefully, and by keeping a lookout for obstructions under
the water. Shoaling water does mean that you need to carefully select channels to paddle at low tides. Even half an hour can make the difference between
completing a passage and being grounded by a mud flat. There are few areas
where a marine chart goes out of date faster than in Glacier Bay, so be sure to
use the newest edition available.

A trip in the Beardslees is ideal for paddlers who want to familiarize themselves with their kayak before embarking on either longer trips, or trips in
more open water. The entire route can be paddled without exposure to significant currents, and without being more than a few hundred yards from shelter in a cove or behind a protecting islet. A trip within the islands is not phys-
ically demanding. Yet the myriad channels and routes which you can paddle
within the Beardslees will give you a real taste of Glacier Bay.

The non-motorized regulation assures kayakers of peace and seclusion
during the majority of the season. Closures to protect wildlife, such as seals
and nesting birds, are imposed for certain areas within the islands, and must
be observed by kayakers. Closure areas in 1997 were Spider, Eider, Flapjack,
Strawberry and the south one-half of South Marble islands.

There are black bears on many of the islands. Since these animals can swim
freely between the islands, protect your food and exercise care to minimize
odors. Moose are also common on the larger islands. You can expect to see
them very early and late in the day when they are grazing on rye grass along
the shore.

While the trip narrative describes a specific route winding through the
islands, the choice is admittedly an arbitrary one. Your own choice of routes
might be just as enjoyable as the one described here. Many different routes
and side explorations are possible, each providing opportunities to experience
the islands and the scenery. You may want to use the following route as a way
to get into, and out of, the islands, while fully exploring as many of the waterways, coves and islands as possible.

Trip Description

Put your boat in the water at the Park Service dock in Bartlett Cove (Map 1), stow your gear aboard, and start paddling. You are already in Beardslee Island waters. After a few minutes of paddling, the initial adrenal rush of finally getting started wears off, and you can look around.

The island forming the opposite shore of Bartlett Cove, directly to the north, is Lester Island, largest of the group. The route leads northeast, around the east end of Lester Island. If possible, plan to paddle the channel between the island and mainland during slack water at high tide. This will give you a reasonable amount of time before strong currents affect the channel. If you wait too long after slack water, when the tide is ebbing, this channel will go dry. If you are in the middle when this happens, it will mean a long wait for the water to return.

At 0.5 mile from the dock, you pass Lagoon Island on your right. You round the east end of Lester Island 1 mile after Lagoon. Now a cove, some 0.5 mile deep, opens up on your right. The Bartlett River enters here. Two small islands, which are not wooded as is the shore of the cove behind them, occupy the center of the bay. Unfortunately, much of this cove turns to mud at low tide, except for the Bartlett River channel.

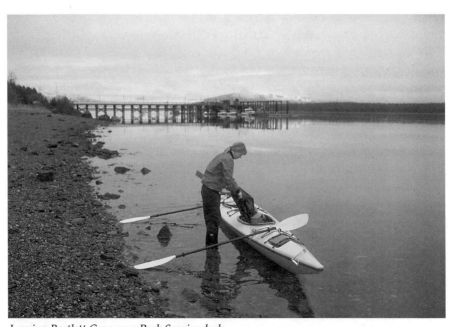

Leaving Bartlett Cove near Park Service dock

The route leads northwest from the cove, passing between an east point of Lester Island some 0.7 mile ahead and an opposing mainland point several hundred yards away to the east. Just past the points, a narrow waterway leading eastward is shown on your chart. Rising land has dried out this passage, and the former island on your right is now a peninsula.

Watch for black oystercatchers here, working along the shore on your left. Lester Island does not offer favorable campsites along this shore. Even if a spot looks good at high tide, the gently sloping, muddy bottom could necessitate a long hike to launch when the tide is out.

Continue on a northwest heading from the dry passage, and paddle near a point of mainland to the east in 0.5 mile. Soon you pass on your left a channel which separates Lester and the neighboring island to the north, but which is only bare rocks and mud at low tide. Leaving Lester Island behind, you head due north opposite a small, 0.5-mile-long island on the west. From the 0.5-mile-long island, a paddle of 2.7 miles on a heading just east of north will take you near the center of Hutchins Bay. Here glacial gouging resulted in the deepest water in the Beardslee group, just over 200 feet deep. The bottom at that depth is shown on charts as being rocky, suggesting that it may be bedrock, and not overlain with the glacial till and silt that form the Beardslee Islands themselves.

From the center of Hutchins Bay, to your right (east) is a half-mile-long, rounded cove, with a sizable stream running in. The terrain forming the drainage area for this stream is nearly flat; lakes lie along the stream course inland 1.5 miles from the mouth. This is an area favored by black bears. These animals are commonly seen along the mainland shore, as well as on the islands.

To the north is a 2-mile-long fiord-like cove, that is 0.5 mile wide at the mouth but quickly narrows to a few hundred yards. A lake lies in the center of the peninsula forming the west side of this cove. It's outlet stream empties a quarter mile east of the southern end of the peninsula. On topo map Juneau (C-6) the topo survey mark SOLE is located on the southwest point of the peninsula.

Kidney Island forms the southwest shore of Hutchins Bay, and provides several good camping spots from its midriff northward along the east, north, and west shores. Any grassy spot with a view northeast into the Bay Park Wilderness is a good bet. Be sure to select a steeply sloping beach where you will be able to easily return to the water at low tide.

From the north point of Kidney Island, head north, and follow the mainland shore. Soon Link Island will be on your left (west). There are several good campsites on both the east and west sides of Link; sunset views over nearby wooded islands are an added bonus on the west side. Between Link and the mainland are rocks in the middle of the channel which are layed bare at low tide. Paddle 2 miles north, past two distinct coves along the north shore which penetrate the forest a half mile. Your route will curve west around the north end of Link Island.

Just a few years ago, there was a choice of two routes at this location. This choice is probably shown on your chart. Northwest 0.5 mile from the north end of Link Island, a narrow passage is shown as leading north into Beartrack Cove. Unfortunately, this channel is no longer passable. Rising land has drained this passage, even at high tide.

Beartrack Cove Option

If you want to paddle into Beartrack Cove, this is as good a place as any from which to begin. Paddle past the drained passage, then turn southeast between the mainland and an unnamed island, toward the islet with the topo survey mark SPIDER (10 miles from your put-in at Bartlett Cove). (Do not confuse the survey mark with Spider Island.) Before reaching this islet, turn north and follow the west shore of what is now mainland peninsula approximately 2 miles into Beartrack Cove. Since this passage is exposed at low tide, you may have to wait a short time for the water to return. But it is a pleasant spot, with a long, grassy point jutting out from the west shore to provide possible camping. Millions of mussels color the intertidal zone here.

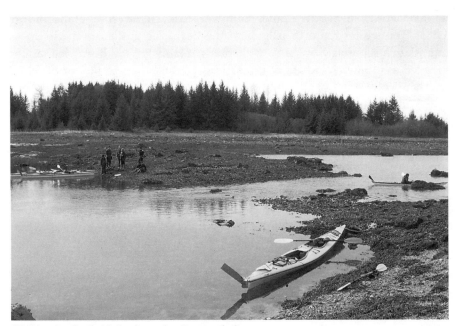

Waiting for flood tide in channel to Beartrack Cove

Beartrack Cove is exposed to the sweep of wind coming down Glacier Bay. Conditions are much less hospitable than among the islands. But if it is blowing, you can always return to the island group through the passage you just negotiated. Assuming the weather is cooperating, paddle through the passage and on into the cove. As soon as you clear the point of the island on your left, you can see 7 miles north along the far shore of Beartrack Cove to South Sandy Cove, the farthest visible landmark. If you are combining Trips 1 and 2, follow the description for Trip 2 from here (12 miles from your put-in at Bartlett Cove).

Three miles closer and to the northwest are the Leland Islands, which appear from this perspective to be a single, narrow island. Still farther west are South and North Marble, small islands about the same distance away as Leland, but only visible from here as rounded white domes. This coloration is due to the limestone forming the islands, which is made even more white by the additional mass of bird guano deposited here.

To return to the Beardslees, go 1.5 miles around the far side of the island which forms the southwest point of Beartrack Cove. Doing so will lead you in a southwest direction through a jumble of small islets at the north end of a group of unnamed islands. At this point, Flapjack Island lies about 1 mile due west. The trip into Beartrack Cove has added about 4 miles to your total route.

—*end of Beartrack Cove Option*

If you don't want to enter Beartrack Cove, head west around the north end of Link Island; then paddle 2 miles southwest to reach the center of the midriff cluster. The western midriff islands of the Beardslee group are made up of nine islands separated by narrow channels. Years ago, the Beardslee family operated a commercial fox farm on the larger island in the center of the cluster. There is little left of this enterprise except a few pilings in a south-shore cove. The fox farm location is shown on topo map Juneau (B-6), but you have little hope of reaching it because of the substantial undergrowth.

The midriff cluster is an excellent place to explore. The channels are narrow, and there are lots of coves through which to paddle. The rapid uplift of the area has caused a nuisance, however. Extensive mud flats are uncovered at low tide. Make sure you are not stranded on a mud flat with the tide ebbing. There is an excellent campsite on the west end of the northernmost islet in this group, just south of the survey mark SWIM on the topo map. Here a startling view of the awesome Fairweather Range will delight the paddler. A sunset from this spot is memorable.

Southwest of this cluster is the Beardslee Entrance, a channel of the main bay with strong currents. Few paddlers visit sizable Strawberry Island, which separates Beardslee Entrance from Sitakaday Narrows. An open crossing of more than a mile is required to reach Strawberry. Unless you are an experienced kayaker or in a capable group, it may be better not to venture to Strawberry Island. Before you go, check for wildlife closures.

From the midriff islands, paddle 1.5 miles southeast to Spider Island, which, at about 0.2 mile long, is the largest of a group of five or six islets. Pass close to Eider Island, 0.7 mile south of Spider (20 miles from Bartlett Cove). Spider, Eider and other islets in this area are frequented by hundreds of sea birds, so do not go ashore on these islands. You may also see concentrations of seals on the rocks in this vicinity. The Park Service closes the area in the vicinity of Spider Island in deference to the seals. Be sure to check closures in effect at the time you plan to paddle. Continue 0.5 mile due south of Eider towards the north shore of a 2-mile-long, unnamed island. Paddle west around that island, through the channel between it and Young Island.

Paddling southeast through this channel leads you into fascinating, calm Secret Bay. This is another excellent area to explore at leisure. Waters are very protected, and currents are light except in the channels during times of mid-flow. The best campsites can be found here, as at other spots in Glacier Bay, by searching in suitable areas that have three or four fathoms of depth close to the shore. Such sites assure that you will be able to come and go with your boat, without wading through acres of mud as the tide goes out. Several good campsites await you in this bay.

From idyllic Secret Bay, you could return to Bartlett Cove by paddling east along the north shore of Lester Island, turning south around its east end, and entering Bartlett Cove by the same route on which you set out. From there it is a 1-mile paddle to the Park Service dock. Just remember that this is a high-tide-only route.

A more adventuresome route leads southeast between Lester and Young Islands. Passable at high tide only, this channel opens out into the large expanse of Glacier Bay just south of Sitakaday Narrows. Strong currents are the rule in the Narrows, so stay close to shore. Some kelp patches offer limited wave protection. From the west end of this channel, paddle east-southeast along the shore of Lester Island; within 1 mile you round a point (27.5 miles from the start) and enter the more placid waters of Bartlett Cove. From the south point of Lester Island, it is a 1.5-mile paddle east to the Park Service dock.

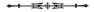

My wife, Laurie, and I leave Bartlett Cove too late, half an hour after high water, and a noticeable current is already running. Against this ebb tide we must make our way into the Beardslees. The excitement of being here at last, kayaking on the waters of Glacier Bay, powers our paddles, and we slide easily through the passage into placid waters.

The islands and islets are as we had imagined, densely forested with trees, presenting an even, sculptured contour. Many of the low-lying islands have few trees, or trees that are not very tall. At first we attribute this to poor soil nutrients; then it slowly dawns that these islands are new. They have only recently become islands due to uplift, and the forest upon them is much younger than upon islands of higher elevations. We are elated to recognize graphic evidence of rapid geologic change in Glacier Bay.

Alders line the shore like a landscape border, as if appointed to separate the high-tide line from the coniferous forest. In many places, salt-tolerant rye grass borders the alders at the extreme high-tide mark. Shore is always nearby, which reinforces our affinity for the land even though we are travelling over water. We slow our synchronized, rhythmic strokes, and let the friendly, peaceful feel of the place sink into our awareness. Halfway between low and high tide we can detect only a gentle tug of currents; the islands divide the movement in all directions.

It is afternoon now, and we know that capricious breezes are whipping the channel just a few miles to the west. But nestled in the protection of the island group, the wind is gentle, coaxing only small ripples on the water through which our sleek boat slips without resistance. Bald eagles look down on us from perches in spruce along the shore. Some flap away ponderously, their wingspans dwarfing those of all other birds in the air. One eagle feeds in the intertidal zone. We decline to approach close enough to identify the meal. A pair of harlequin ducks feed close to shore, keeping an eye on us all the while. The male is in breeding plumage, a kaleidoscope of chestnuts, blacks and whites. A raft of scaup paddle by, the drakes saucy in their black-and-white tuxedos. A haunting, half-human cry comes from a grayish bird some distance away, which binoculars confirm is a red-necked loon. In less than an hour, we spot our first black bear. The animal is across the channel from us, feeding at the edge of the alders on shoots of rye grass. We land on our side and watch the grazing creature for half an hour. The bear pays no attention. As we look, we are further mesmerized by the odd combination of raw wilderness and peaceful welcome; both mark this island group. Later in the day two moose appear, a cow and nearly grown calf, grazing in the rye across the channel. We stop paddling and glass the animals, black, awkward, ugly in any context except in nature where everything is perfectly suited for its niche.

After making camp, we talk about our first day in Glacier Bay. We are happy with our immersion in nature. We have seen pigeon guillemots, their sooty black accented only by white wing bars until they fly. Then brilliant, red-orange feet churn madly along the surface until their flying speed is achieved. Gulls, cormorants, grebes and mergansers have entertained us all day. We have almost grown accustomed to the smooth, round heads of the harbor seals, bobbing at the surface, whose sad eyes watch our passage.

We stash our bearproof food containers some distance from the tent, and turn in. The dulling concerns of our ordinary life have slipped away and are not missed. The sun blazes orange, then, in the final moments, fractures through spruce limbs into rays. The glow remains for a long time, and true darkness does not come.

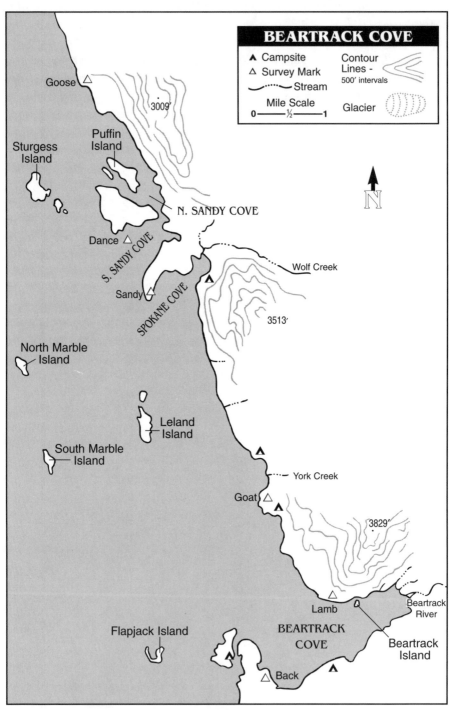

BEARTRACK COVE

▲ Campsite
△ Survey Mark
‿‿‿ Stream
Mile Scale
0 ——— ½ ——— 1

Contour
Lines -
500' intervals

Glacier

Goose △
3009'

Puffin
Island

Sturgess
Island

N. SANDY COVE

Dance △

S. SANDY COVE

Sandy △

SPOKANE COVE

Wolf Creek

3513'

North Marble
Island

Leland
Island

South Marble
Island

York Creek

Goat △

3829'

Lamb △

Beartrack
River

BEARTRACK
COVE

Beartrack
Island

Flapjack Island

Back △

N

MAP 2

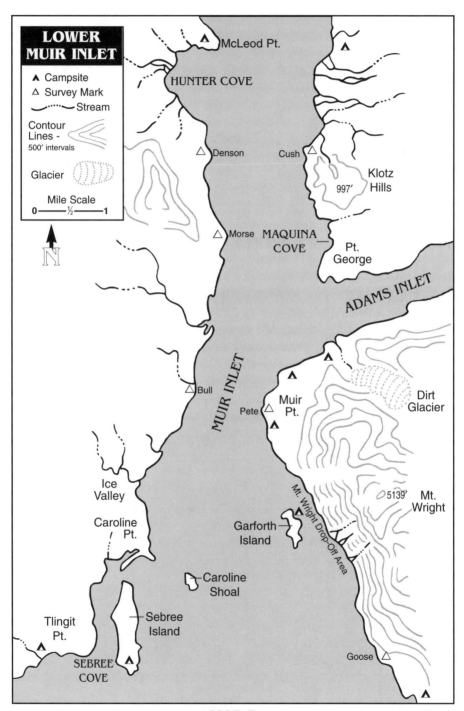

McLeod Pt.

HUNTER COVE

Denson

Cush

Klotz
Hills

997'

Morse

MAQUINA
COVE

Pt.
George

ADAMS INLET

MUIR INLET

Bull

Pete

Muir
Pt.

Dirt
Glacier

Ice
Valley

5139'

Mt.
Wright

Caroline
Pt.

Garforth
Island

Mt. Wright Drop-Off Area

Caroline
Shoal

Tlingit
Pt.

Sebree
Island

Goose

SEBREE
COVE

MAP 3

Chapter 6

TRIP 2   MT. WRIGHT TO BEARTRACK COVE

Trip Details

Distance:	47 miles RT from Mt. Wright drop-off
	42 miles one way from Mt. Wright drop-off to Bartlett Cove
	20 miles one way from Beartrack Cove to Mt. Wright pickup
Time:	5-7 days
Rating:	Moderate
Maps:	NOAA Chart 17318; USGS Topos: Juneau (C-6), Mt. Fairweather (C-1) & (D-1)

Summary and Highlights

In this trip you visit offshore islands, experience secluded coves, and are in close proximity to bird rookeries and a sea lion haulout spot. Humpbacks frequently feed in the area from the Sandy Coves north to Garforth Island, but the whale-waters classification does not restrict kayakers. Puffin Island provides nesting sites for tufted puffins during early summer. Mountain goats are commonly seen along the shoreline, especially on the slopes of Mt. Wright. Black bears are frequent visitors to the intertidal areas bordering this route, especially early in the season when they are feeding on grass shoots and mollusks. Bear closures in 1997 extended from Wolf Creek in Spokane Cove, north to the south tip of Garforth Island, from May 1 through August 15. Check for any changes to the closures at park headquarters prior to your trip. There is good camping in several places on this trip, particularly between Beartrack Cove and the Sandy Coves. Camping along the closed section farther north is limited to offshore islands.

Hazards: Very cold water is a hazard to kayakers. The trip as described involves crossing Beartrack Cove, an exposed, open-water paddle of 1.6 miles, on the return trip to Mt. Wright. Similarly, the east coast of Glacier Bay bordering the trip route is open water, unprotected from winds from the north or northwest. Wind waves can develop rapidly.

Area Features, Background, and Tips

Beartrack Cove lies at the northern end of the Beardslee Islands, and presents the northbound paddler with the first taste of open, exposed water. Wind direction during periods of clear weather is often from the north, where the wind can blow for 20 miles across open water. You need to take the wind strength into account when paddling in this area, particularly in the afternoon.

The Beartrack River flows into the head of Beartrack Cove. Around 15 miles in length, it drains an area of several dozen square miles north of the cove and as far east as the divide at the park boundary. Streams of this size mean food for bears, especially during salmon spawning season. You will probably see tracks as well as the bears themselves on this trip. Large inflow streams also indicate widespread tidal flats, which exist along the east and north shores of the cove.

Beartrack Island, halfway into the cove near the north shore, is an island at high water only. During low tides, it is connected to the mainland by mud flats. Campsites along the south shore of the cove are not recommended because they are exposed to the prevailing wind. Campsites do exist on the north shore, just west of Beartrack Island.

Since Beartrack Cove was free of ice by 1820, adequate time has elapsed for a respectable forest to grow. The shoreline is densely wooded with conifers that have shaded out the alders and cottonwoods. Paddling up this coast, you will notice the diminishing size of the coniferous forest.

Many paddlers spend time on the protected beach one mile south of York Creek (near GOAT survey marker). A blunt point provides shelter, and a series of older gravel beaches extend varying distances from the water, at different elevations. It is easy to find a campsite above the high water. The alder screen is thin to nonexistent here. On entering the forest you are immediately engulfed in a moss-carpeted rain forest where devil's club spreads its broad, spiny leaves. Bear trails lace the moss in every direction. York Creek drains a small glacier 5 miles inland, as well as other ice fields. The final outpouring to salt water is tumultuous, roaring over and around granite boulders. From this point northward, campsites are scarce and limited.

Northwest of York Creek, Leland Island dominates the view of Glacier Bay. Some 5 miles offshore beyond it, are South Marble and North Marble islands. South Marble's southern half is closed year around, including the waters within 50 yards of shore. This island is a common haul-out spot for sea lions, and the only place within Glacier Bay where these animals are found. Both North and South Marble islands are bird rookeries. The Park Service recommends not going ashore on any unwooded islands to avoid disturbing birds which primarily congregate and nest on bare rock. Both Marble Islands are easily recognized at a distance by their distinctive dome shape, lack of vegetation, and near-white, bird-guano and natural limestone coloring. A visit to the proximity of these islands should be considered only during times of calm water because of their distance from shore.

Wolf Creek is one of two streams entering at the head of Spokane Cove. Both streams drain several square miles of territory. Extensive tidal flats dominate the east end of the cove, flanked by dense stands of rye grass, and alders.

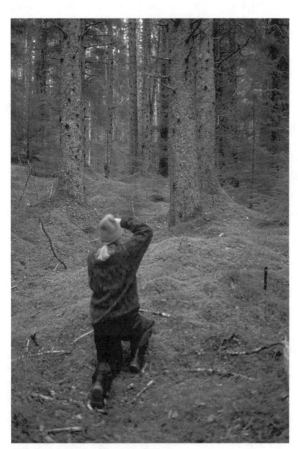

Rainforest north of Beartrack Cove

In the early spring, it is hard to imagine more perfect bear habitat. The closure area due to bear activity begins at Wolf Creek. After bear-closure restrictions are lifted, there is good camping along the north shore of the peninsula enclosing Spokane Cove. The best is near the blunt point forming the north shore at the mouth of the cove proper. Be sure to pick a campsite above high water, where adequate water depth exists near shore to avoid stranding your kayak.

South Sandy Cove offers great protection from all winds except strong westerlies. The island shown as the topo survey mark DANCE becomes the tip of a small peninsula at low water.

Inside its shelter and that furnished by other points, the water is usually calm. The passage between South and North Sandy coves is dry except at high tide, so using this narrow time slot requires careful attention to the tides.

Whether the main feature of North Sandy Cove is Puffin Island, or the delightful mini-bay that lies at its east end, is up to the individual. Puffin Island sports many cliffs, colorful lichens and rocks, and is home to easily observed tidal creatures such as stars and chitons. In the summer it also hosts nesting tufted puffins. Nest sites in rock jumbles and cracks in cliffs can sometimes be identified by the dirt which the birds have excavated from their nesting burrows. Within the mini-bay, about a half square mile in area, are a variety of shorelines—cliffs and grassy flats—tiny coves, various bird habitats, and most important, completely protected water. These benefits attract small cruise ships which frequently anchor here. Such "eco-tour" passengers are good neighbors, but their presence can be disconcerting to kayakers who have paddled many miles in search of wilderness and solitude.

From Puffin Island 4 miles north to Mt. Wright, there is little protection offered along shore. Two distinct points within the first mile and a half can shelter you from northerly breezes. Beyond that, only tiny coves and points provide less-than-ideal shelter. The shoreline becomes especially precipitous along the west slopes of Mt. Wright. Northbound paddlers caught in windy conditions along this section can consider stopping at Garforth Island, which is less than half a mile from the mainland shore. Camping is possible near the north and south ends of the island. Fortunately, Glacier Bay narrows as you approach the entrance to Muir Point, reducing the wind's sweep.

Trip Description

If you are making Trip 2 as a continuation of Trip 1, paddle this trip route in reverse (northbound). This trip begins at the Mt. Wright drop-off point, on the mainland shore east of Garforth Island (Map 3). From the Mt. Wright drop-off, paddle 2 miles south to a sizable stream. South of this stream the shoreline, previously bare, becomes wooded. Go 1 mile south of the stream to a small point, topo survey mark GOOSE, which provides shelter from northerly winds and waves (Map 2). Continue 1 mile south of GOOSE to a distinct point offering protection in its lee.

Camping here is possible after the bear closure ends on August 15. There are limited camping sites along this shore; just where you pitch a tent depends upon whether winter storms have removed or deposited gravel on beaches in coves and at points. If sufficient gravel is present in front of the sloping rock confines of these coves or points, campsites can easily be made above the high-water mark.

From the sheltering point it is an easy 1-mile paddle south to the north end of Puffin Island. From the north end, continue 1 mile south along the east

shore of Puffin. Clear water and good conditions here insure lots of interesting life among the rocks in the intertidal zone. You may see the nesting sites
of the tufted puffin. At the south end of Puffin Island is the delightful head of
North Sandy Cove. Explore its east and south shores, where tiny, tucked-away
coves insure intimacy in these very sheltered waters. Along a section of the
shore, grassy flats provide grazing for black bears making their rounds in the
early spring.

A narrow passage at the south end of North Sandy Cove may lead to South
Sandy Cove during higher tides. The more reliable route leads northwest.
Paddle 1 mile along the west shore of Puffin Island to a tiny, narrow islet that
lies just yards off the west side of Puffin. Turn west, rounding the north end
of the islet; then paddle 1.5 miles south to the entrance of South Sandy Cove.
During low water, it is best to stay south of the islet with the topo survey mark
DANCE before turning east and continuing 1 mile to the head of South Sandy
Cove.

From South Sandy Cove, head 1.5 miles southwest around the point with
the topo survey mark SANDY, then paddle 1.5 miles east to the headwaters of
Spokane Cove (13 miles from the Mt. Wright drop-off). Camping restrictions
end on the north shore of Wolf Creek, flowing into Spokane Cove. Camping
possibilities exist in a small bight southeast of the cove, if you believe that the
bears respect their closure boundaries and do not cross Wolf Creek. After the
camping closure ends, the better sites are found along the north shore of the
peninsula, southwest of the cove.

From Spokane Cove, you can visit Leland Island, and perhaps North and
South Marble islands if conditions are calm. North Marble Island lies 4.5 miles
west southwest of the head of Spokane Cove. This open-water crossing is
hedged somewhat by Leland Island, about 1.5 miles south of the midway
point. South Marble Island is 2 miles south of its northern sister. Open-water
crossings of this nature should be undertaken with caution after assessing
both the weather conditions and your capabilities.

Paddle 4 miles south from Spokane Cove to York Creek. The shoreline along
this section is characterized by slopes rising steeply from the water to elevations of 1000 feet. Camping between Spokane Cove and York Creek is extremely limited, as is shelter. A small, jutting point just north of York Creek offers
camping and protection from the waves. Be aware that there is a shallow, submerged rock just off this point. Landing is easy on a gravel beach just south of
the stream mouth in York Creek Cove. A great camping area exists 0.5 mile
south of the topo survey mark GOAT. Several fine gravel beaches offer choice
spots. In early season, water is often available near the east end of the beach.

From York Creek, paddle 3.5 miles south to the topo survey mark LAMB.
From LAMB, paddle 1.5 miles east into the head of Beartrack Cove. Beartrack
Island, on the north shore of the cove, marks the beginning of tidal flats which

extend to the head of the cove and south of the inflow of the Beartrack River. The north shoreline slopes steeply to nearly 4000 feet, while the south and east shores of the cove are almost flat, rising little more than 100 feet two miles inland. From the head of Beartrack Cove, paddle 3 miles southwest along the south shore to the heel of the cove. Watch for submerged rocks along this shoreline. The small coves in this area invite exploration, but remember that many will become mud flats at low water. Your chart may indicate a channel through to the Beardslee Islands here, but at normal water levels this passage is dry.

From the small coves, go 1.5 miles northwest, past the point with the topo survey mark BACK, to a passage leading south between the peninsula to your left, and the island just west of it. This spot marks the end of the trip described in this chapter (27 miles from the Mt. Wright drop-off).

From this point, you may end the paddle by continuing 15 miles south through the Beardslee Islands to Bartlett Cove as described in Chapter 5 (Trip 1). Alternatively, paddle north and return to the Mt. Wright pickup point. Excluding the cove side trips described on the southbound route, the Mt. Wright pickup point is 20 miles away.

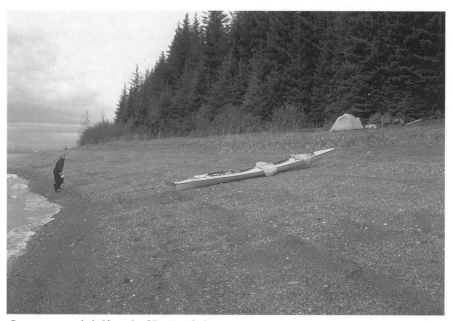

Camp on gravel shelf north of Beartrack Cove

We intended to slip into Beartrack Cove from the Beardslees through the narrow channel between their northernmost island and the peninsula to the east. Helped by a flood tide, we did fine until encountering a dry spot in mid-channel. Millions of mussels, forming a royal blue-purple carpet in the intertidal zone, lent visual stimulation as we waited. A first trickle of water ran its rivulet across the reef of mussels, quickly becoming a stream deep enough to float our kayak. We paddled a tiny, secondary bay, and entered Beartrack Cove.

Afternoons are not the best time for open crossings, and this afternoon a 10-knot wind, sweeping from the north across 20 miles of open water, kicked up 18-inch waves. We quartered into the waves, and crossed the 2-mile width of Beartrack Cove to the north shore. The shoreline offered us some protection. Turning north, we paddled up the coast to a welcome campsite at the inland end of a south-facing beach one mile below York Creek. Snug from the wind and yet tired from the paddle, we set up camp on the highest gravel shelf, above all visible signs of high water. Our stove hissed while we anchored the tent, then moved the boat above high water, and tied it to alders. After hot food and drinks on the beach, we relaxed to write in our logs as a light sprinkle fell on the tent.

Morning brought a steely sky and unabated wind. Anxious as we were to see more of this coast, little was to be gained by paddling directly into a minor gale. By ten o'clock, the wind diminished and we were able to head north. York Creek descended in a rush of whitewater as it entered the bay. There was wildlife here. A pair of especially bright harlequin ducks paddled out of our way as we landed to replenish drinking water. A blue heron peered at us with suspicion before taking wing. Brilliant green algae affixed to granite boulders below the high-tide line contrasted with the foaming white water.

Intrigued by Leland Island just 2 miles west, we considered the camping possibilities there. All but the south tip of the island is closed to landing year around. When we looked into Spokane Cove, 3 miles north, our binoculars revealed a couple of black bears grazing just above the high-tide mark. Homing on the tiny black dots, we paddled nearer for half an hour. The hooked peninsula jutting southwest between Spokane and South Sandy coves stopped the wind, and our boat slipped over the calm surface like a knife. We spotted more bears ashore, and, mindful of the bear closure in effect here, changed course to round the peninsula, leaving Spokane Cove to its ursine occupants.

The exposed rock faces on Puffin Island presented lichens and colors markedly different from the shoreline to the south. We paddled close to the island, speculating on which fissure or crack provided nesting sites to tufted puffins. Drifting very close to the island, we saw many chitons and sea stars clinging to rocks in the intertidal zone at the base of cliffs.

The wide, protected east end of North Sandy Cove is a kayaker's dream. We spotted another kayak in the cove, and as we rounded the point, a 200' cruise vessel came into view. Anchored there, the ship gave passengers a taste of the intimate coves of Glacier Bay. As we watched, a dozen kayaks were launched to paddle in the cove. A black bear on shore drew much attention.

As we left this reminder of civilization behind and headed north, a white dot moving far up on a precipitous slope caught our eye. Our first mountain goat scouted for several more that came into view on the high cliffs. For a minute we drifted in our kayak, watching. A feeling of belonging settled over us. Careful not to break the spell, we dipped our paddles and headed north.

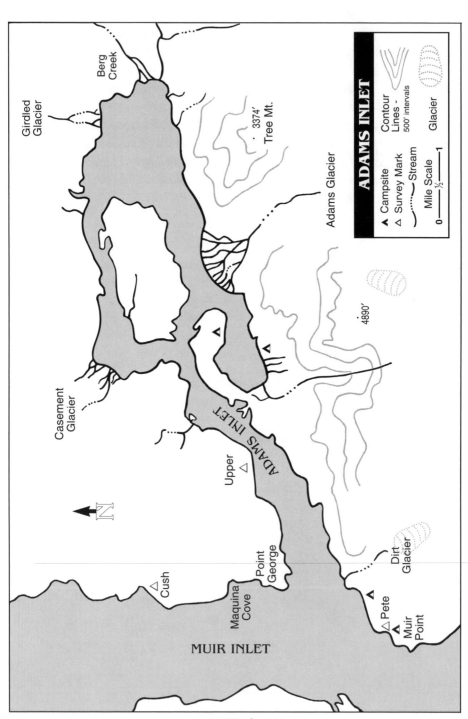

MAP 4

Chapter 7

TRIP 3 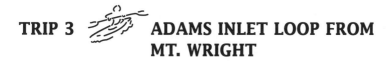 **ADAMS INLET LOOP FROM MT. WRIGHT**

Trip Details

Distance:	27 miles RT from Mt. Wright drop-off
	21 miles RT from inlet entrance
Time:	3-6 days
Rating:	Easy to Moderate
Maps:	NOAA Chart 17318; USGS Topos: Juneau (D-6), Mt. Fairweather (D-1)

Summary and Highlights

Adams Inlet is a birdwatcher's paradise. Moraines, glacial outwash, and Endicott Gap (portal for land mammals repopulating the Muir Inlet area after the ice melted) are evident to the paddler. Good-to-excellent camping, and fresh water, can be found at several locations. The inlet is a terrific destination for a one-week paddle utilizing the drop-off services provided by the concessionaire to the Mt. Wright location. Daily drop-off time is around 9:00 A.M. Concessionaire contact data is found in the Appendix.

Adams Inlet is presently is classified as non-motorized water from May 15 through September 15. Whether this motor-vessel closure is responsible for the abundant bird life seen here is not clear. Kayakers benefit by enjoying this stunning inlet—camping and paddling here—most of the season without disturbance from motorized boats.

Hazards: Cold water, winds, and currents are ever-present dangers to kayakers in northern waters. No exposed crossings are necessary to make this trip. Strong currents can be present at times 2 miles east of the entrance in Adams Inlet.

Area Features, Background, and Tips

The Muir Inlet arm branches north from Glacier Bay 35 miles from the bay mouth. Within 3 miles, Muir Inlet narrows to slightly more than one mile in width. In 2 more miles 10-mile-long Adams Inlet lies to the east. Adams is spectacular because of the plentiful bird life to be seen here, perhaps more than at other estuaries within Glacier Bay.

Little of the shore rises abruptly from the water. The large island in the center of the inlet is very low, covered with cottonwood and alder. The same is true of the nearly 2-milelong, curved peninsula which lies west of the inflow from Adams Glacier. While the sharp north slope of Tree Mountain at the southeast end of the inlet does plunge into tidewater, the remainder of Adams Inlet's shore is gentle in slope. This, of course, is the result of alluvial action and sedimentation which is quite rapidly filling the inlet. Add the effects of uplift, and it is anyone's guess how many decades will pass before the inlet is no longer navigable.

The narrow entrance channel which funnels large water volumes contained in the easternmost expanse of the inlet does generate currents capable of scouring out accumulated sediments. But processes are at work which will ultimately cause the inlet to become a stagnant backwater, or one large delta for the glacial streams. The narrow channel north of the large, unnamed island reveals mudflats during ebb tides. This occurs around 10 feet above mean low water.

Contrasting with the dense vegetation on the island and much of the shoreline, is the relatively bare outwash fan from Adams Glacier. Paddle near the mouth of the muddy stream and you can hear the water moving larger particles and rocks along the bottom, constantly building the fan outward. Since this fan is new land, only a few, early colonizing plants exist on it. In fact, most of the dense vegetation in Adams Inlet is relatively new, consisting mostly of alder and cottonwood, both fairly early occupants in the chain of succession.

While extensive mud flats are visible at all times except high water, there are several, excellent camping areas within the inlet. Water can always be found in the major melt streams, but such flows carry silt. Yet, a few, clear, snow-melt streams are found on the slopes of Tree Mountain, even late in the season. Some of the better campsites have clear streamlets nearby. Other sites within the inlet must be considered dry, and you should carry water.

Streams flowing into Adams Inlet at its eastern end originate in a low divide, or pass. The Endicott River drains the slope east of the divide, emptying into Lynn Canal. The Southeast Alaska towns of Haines and Skagway lie on small inlets at the northern end of Lynn Canal. Because of the low elevation of this divide, and the fact that the Lynn Canal side was free of ice centuries before the Glacier Bay side, the pass was the natural route through which land mammals entered Glacier Bay drainages once the ice melted.

Trip Description

Trip 3 may be done as described, or done as a continuation of Trip 4. From the Mt. Wright drop-off point, paddle north along the east shore entrance to Muir Inlet (Map 3). Garforth Island lies 0.3 mile off the shore to the west. North of Garforth Island, the mainland shore changes from steep cliffs and ledges to the more heavily wooded flats of Muir Point. If you intend to camp in the Muir Point area, collect water from one of the small streams draining the west slope of Mt. Wright.

Muir Point is 2 miles north of Garforth Island. There are many possible campsites here and it is easy to land almost anywhere. Make sure the site you choose is above the high-tide mark. The extensive growth of rye grass along this shore can obscure signs of high water. Muir Point beaches consist of gravel or small boulders, and slope abruptly so that putting in during low water is not difficult. There is also a good camping beach in a small cove about 0.2 mile west of the outflow from Dirt Glacier (4 miles from the Mt. Wright drop-off). Here, too, it is easy to land and camp above high tide, but there is no water. Whether you are visiting Adams Inlet from the drop-off point on Mt. Wright, or are on a longer trip, the Muir Point area is a great place to camp and wait for a favorable tide to enter Adams Inlet. Entering the inlet as the flood tide begins will assure an easy paddle, so you can take your time here and let the sometimes considerable current do part of the work there.

Leave the Dirt Glacier camp behind, and head east into Adams Inlet (Map 4). You will pass the Dirt Glacier melt stream, and while you may hear the water, you cannot see the glacier. It is hidden up the canyon, more than a mile away from tidewater. Just east of this stream are two small islands, which will blend in with and become part of a mudflat at low tide. Keep an eye out for moose on both shores of the Adams Inlet entrance and channel. As big as they are, these animals blend in easily with shore rocks and vegetation; so, binoculars are a great help. Excellent moose habitat exists along the north entrance, east of Point George.

About 2 miles east of the two islets is an unmistakable cove on the south shore. Again, extensive mud flats at low water make this an unpractical camping spot (6 miles from the Mt. Wright drop-off). From this cove paddle northeast diagonally across Adams Inlet toward that point with the topo survey mark UPPER. Rocks and shoals in this section of the channel concentrate the current, which can boil and churn with force during maximum flow. Stay to the north side of the channel. Once you're beyond UPPER, the flow is not as restricted, and the current eases. Harbor seals and porpoise

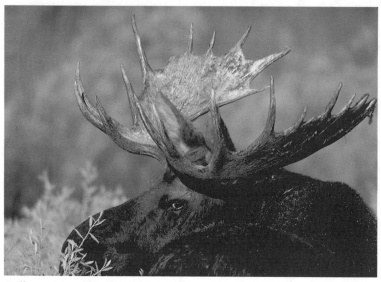

Bull moose in willows

congregate in this channel section to catch the fish lured here by current-borne food.

Along the south shore 1 mile east of UPPER, there are numerous small finger bays which may be dry at low water, but make interesting exploring when depths are sufficient. The land at the head of these bays forms the thin neck of a curving peninsula which will be on your right for the next 2 miles. It's hard to distinguish the profile of this peninsula from that of the large island beyond it. You are now well into the inlet. The smells are less marine, and more estuarine. You begin to notice more bird life from this point on. The channel is narrow here, and for the remainder of your time in the inlet you will never be far from shore.

When you are 1.7 miles northeast from the finger bays, the large, wooded island is directly east, in front of you. To your left a narrow channel runs directly north, later curving east to encircle the island. You could enter the larger, eastern portion of Adams Inlet via this channel. Instead, choose to continue right, along the peninsula, because the main current runs through here and will help you along. A short distance into this southeast reach, a tiny finger bay branches right. You will likely hear the runoff stream from Adams Glacier as you approach the bay south of the channel. Tons of sediment are deposited daily at the Adams outwash. Because of the wealth of nutrients here, watch for the variety of bird life which you can see.

A small bay, with good water depth, lies to the south and west of you. There is excellent camping at several points along the south shore of the bay, with drinking-water streamlets except at the driest times. And, there are some acceptable campsites across the bay on the peninsula. A sizable meltwater stream is building a gravel fan at the west end of this bay. Visiting the west end is worth the paddle. The shoreline is relatively unvegetated, and limited hiking can be done here (10 miles from the Mt. Wright drop-off). Directly south of the bay, and just 1.7 miles away, is a 4890' peak, flanked by snowfields.

From the west end of the bay paddle east toward the Adams Glacier outwash fan. Notice that there is little vegetation on the gravel fan. This is because much of the surface is newly deposited, and sufficient time has not passed for larger plants to grow. Also, frequent course changes of the outflow stream inundate new areas and erode new surfaces.

Upstream, to the south, lies what appears to be a sandy, flat-topped butte with sparse vegetation and steep, exposed soil sides. This is a moraine, deposited by the glacier, and now being eroded away by water forces. The gravel fan is an interesting place to walk, with enough gravel and stone to limit the presence of quicksand, but be careful anyway. Scattered before you are rocks and sand, the results of centuries of grinding, scouring, and tearing by Adams Glacier. From tidewater it is more than 5 miles to the glacier itself, a fairly tough hike that should be reserved for those with experience and high motivation.

The Adams outflow stream may exit anywhere from the east to the west side of the fan, as its course is constantly changing. Continue 2.5 miles east from the fan to a prominent stream flowing down the north face of Tree Mountain. You may see mountain goats on its slopes in this area. At the Berg Creek outflow, 1 mile east, is an extensive mud flat that marks the eastern end of Adams Inlet.

The Berg Creek outflow (14 miles from the Mt. Wright drop-off) is actually the combination of two streams draining the west slope of a low divide. The Endicott River drains the east slope, flowing into the Lynn Canal. The divide, sometimes called Endicott Gap, was the first ice-free route into the land areas around Glacier Bay. Moose, mountain goat, and other land mammals migrated into the bay through this portal soon after the ice receded. They apparently still do, as many tracks of moose, goat, bear, and wolf are commonly seen in the mud flats in this area.

Paddle 1 mile north of the Berg Creek outflow to the Girdled Glacier outwash. Good examples of interstadial stumps, buried by ice for thousands of years, are exposed about 2 miles up the Girdled Glacier outflow stream. The hike to them has become increasingly difficult because of the growth of alders. There are some marginal campsites in the vicinity of the Girdled Glacier outflow, though none are as good as those on the south side of the inlet.

From the Girdled Glacier outflow, head west to the east end of the large island. There are extensive shallows here, and the area may expose mud flats at lower tides. Continue west, along the north side of the island, passing a small, narrow, outrigger island. A short distance beyond it a hammerhead peninsula extends from the island's north shore. There is marginal camping on the handle of the peninsula, but there's no water supply (16 miles from the Mt. Wright drop-off). A large glacial "erratic," a huge boulder carried by glacial ice, was deposited here as the ice melted. It is a conspicuous, rectangular block sitting on an otherwise quite even shoreline.

The north channel around the island should only be used at high water. It goes dry in several places, and can leave you beached for many hours awaiting the water's return. A tide level of 12 feet above mean low water should allow passage at this time. The outwash from Casement Glacier lies 2 miles east of the hammerhead peninsula on the north shore. This, too, is a rapidly changing shoreline, with unreliable depths on your chart. What is shown as a bay will end up mostly being mud flats at low water in the Casement Glacier area. Stay in the middle of the apparent channel when opposite the Casement Glacier outflow. Turn south around the west end of the island, and paddle 1 mile to rejoin the main channel (19 miles from the Mt. Wright drop-off).

Follow the main channel west to where you entered, at the small cove just west of the Dirt Glacier outflow. The return route leads southwest from Dirt Glacier south around Muir Point, then south along shore to the Mt. Wright pickup point (27 miles round trip).

⊷ ⊷ ⧉◆⧈ ⊶ ⊶

It is snug in our tent, warm and dry even though a patter on the fly serves notice that last night's rain still lingers. Now, in the half-light of very early morning, we are anxious to get going.

Our camp is at the entrance to Adams Inlet, in a small cove just west of the Dirt Glacier outflow. Yesterday afternoon, when rounding Muir Point, we had wanted to camp there, near where the famed naturalist built a cabin. But several black bears, grazing and feeding in the intertidal area at quarter-mile intervals, kept us paddling until a mile of beach without bears separated us. We had pitched our tent on sand above the high-water mark.

Low tide had been at 2:47 A.M., and we wanted to ride the flood into Adams Inlet. By 5:00 A.M. a break in the showers allowed us to get the tent down, and camp stowed in the boat. The air was still and damp as we pushed off and headed east into the inlet, ignoring the tiny rings dimpling the glassy surface, reminders that rain still figured into the day. But paddling jackets and snug cockpits are antidotes for most bad weather, and on a 1-knot current, we swept eastward into Adams Inlet. A cow moose and her yearling calf grazed on the north shore just inside the inlet. *Looking from a distance, we made no disturbance to their unhurried munching of rye-grass stalks.*

We quickly passed the Dirt Glacier inflow, with the glacier itself invisibly entrenched in a narrow canyon some distance from tidewater. The current speed increased as the channel narrowed to a few hundred yards. Surface eddies marked the location of mid-channel rocks just south of the survey mark Upper on the north shore point. Cormorants and mergansers flew by, singly and in groups. The sky lightened and the rain stopped, motivating several swallows to practice their erratic, aerial feeding above our heads. As if on cue, Adams Inlet wildlife began to put on a show.

Harlequin ducks in pairs, rafts of greater scaup, and pairs of northern shoveler and mallards all paraded for us. Pigeon guillemots on the water merely paddled out of our way and watched as we passed. Bird sounds noticeably increased, in contrast to the frequent silence of larger water bodies. Harbor seals were constantly bobbing where boils marked underwater rocks and reefs. Black dorsals were emerging and submerging in slow motion; harbor porpoise, too, were taking advantage of the tidal-current lunch counter. Adams Inlet was displaying its own, particular ambiance.

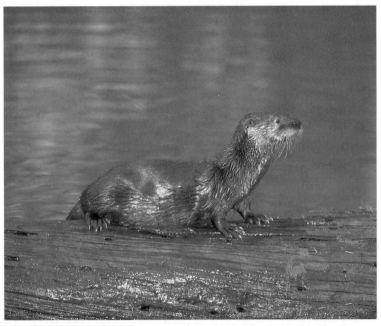

River otter bounds along the estuary shore

From that point on, we were never without Adams Inlet creatures in view. A river otter bounded along shore before abandoning its characteristic land gait for a smooth, watery glide, now reflecting tentative sunshine from its V-wake. Near the large outwash from Adams Glacier, flocks of Canada geese passed noisily overhead. Gulls concentrated here, feeding in the water and resting ashore. Glaucous-winged, mew, and Bonaparte's gulls were thick in the air around our boat. A few, dark-phase parasitic jaegers worried the gulls in hope of a meal. Arctic terns alternately rejoined the melee, and darted out to perform Kamikaze dives for small fish.

Several snow-melt cataracts lined the north slope of Tree Mountain right down to tidewater, the combined music of their rapid fall turning to a roar as we drew closer. Two mountain goats watched unconcerned, 100 feet above tidewater, as we paddled slowly by. Like sentinels they appraised, then dismissed, us as not significant. They had resumed browsing before we had gone far. There is an aura, an ambiance, and a not-unwelcome, inhuman din here. For those seeking a fauna-filled inlet with the noticeable push and pull of tidal currents, Adams Inlet is not disappointing.

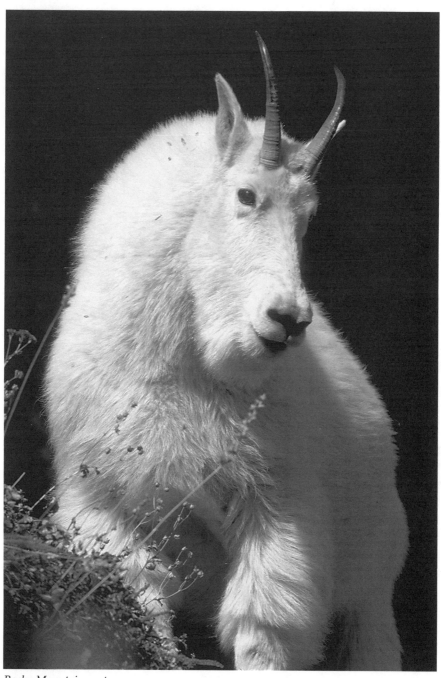

Rocky Mountain goat

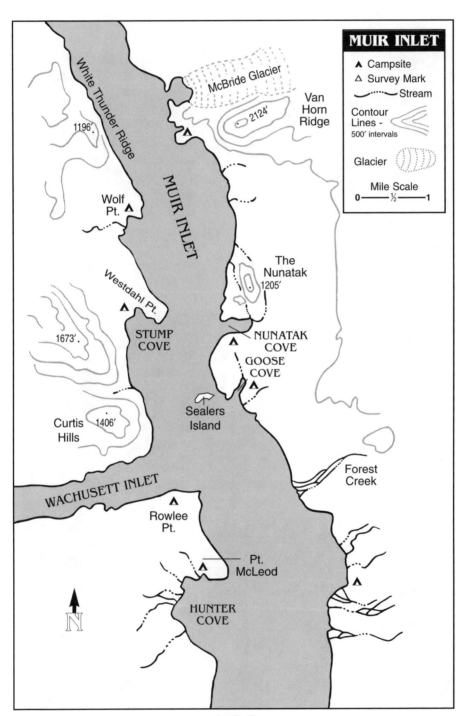

MAP 5

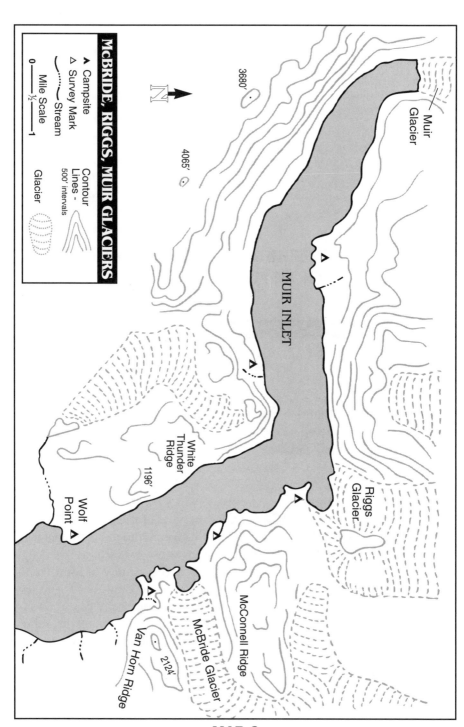

MAP 6

McBRIDE, RIGGS, MUIR GLACIERS

▲ Campsite
△ Survey Mark
Stream

Contour
Lines -
500' intervals

Glacier

Mile Scale
0 — ½ — 1

N

3680'

4065'

Muir
Glacier

MUIR INLET

White
Thunder
Ridge

1196'

Wolf
Point

Riggs
Glacier

McConnell Ridge

McBride Glacier

Van Horn Ridge

2124'

Chapter 8

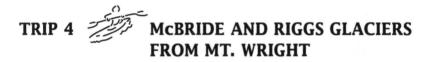

TRIP 4   McBRIDE AND RIGGS GLACIERS FROM MT. WRIGHT

Trip Details

Distance:	34 miles RT from Mt. Wright drop-off
	26 miles RT from Point George
Time:	4-6 days
Rating:	Easy to Moderate
Maps:	NOAA Chart 17318; USGS Topos: Mt. Fairweather (D-1); Skagway (A-3) & (A-4)

Summary and Highlights

This trip visits McBride and Riggs Glaciers, two of the three, major tidewater glaciers in Muir Inlet. Kayaking here brings you into direct contact with icebergs, especially in McBride Lagoon. Harbor seals give birth to their pups on ice floes in this lagoon during early summer. The vicinity of Muir Inlet's Riggs Glacier is closed to motorized vessels from June 1 to July 15. The section of Muir Inlet covered in this trip demonstrates graphically the process of plant succession, beginning with scraggly alder and cottonwood and ending with spruce forest. Striking landforms here include the moraines near Red Mountain, which are being rapidly eroded. Hazards include the ever-present cold water, the possibility of wind and waves in Muir Inlet, and icebergs, especially in the McBride Lagoon.

Area Features, Background, and Tips

The portion of Muir Inlet covered in this trip was freed from the Little Ice Age around 1894 at Adams Inlet, but only released from ice during the mid-1960s at Riggs Glacier. The ice retreated some 15 miles north during this 70-year time span. The characteristic vegetation in the course of the 15-mile paddle reflects this rapid change. Healthy conifer forests at Adams Inlet dwindle to occasional spruce and a few cottonwoods as you go north. By the time McBride Glacier is reached, there are very few conifers. Alder and cottonwood make up the bulk of the vegetation. The young shoreline trees and shrubs add to the feeling of starkness when travelling north to the glaciers, and back to the beginnings of this span of organic life.

This is an easy paddle, particularly along the east shore, except in times of strong winds. Maximum tidal flows are around 1 knot; not serious even if you have to paddle against them. Numerous shoreline features offer shelter from the wind and the waves, no matter whether they're coming from the north or the south.

The scenery constantly assails the senses, making this one of those outstanding paddles. In clear weather, coming from the south, your first view of a glacier is, in fact, not McBride, but Casement Glacier, perched on hills 3 miles northeast of Forest Creek. Casement Glacier does not reach tidewater; its main outflow pours south into Adams Inlet. Views of glaciated knobs, such as The Nunatak, the attending moraines and benches of Red Mountain 3 miles to the east, as well as Van Horn, and McConnell Ridge, hold the interest of kayakers.

Camping is possible along much of the east shore. There are too many coves to mention, most of them with gravel or shingle beaches that invite landing. At most beaches it's easy to locate campsites above high water. Frequent streams supply water along this shore. While most camping is on the east shore, there are good west side camping spots at Wolf Point, Stump Cove, Rowlee Point, and Hunter Cove. The impressive cliffs along White Thunder Ridge offer no camping possibilities. Even landing on talus jumbles there is dangerous because of the possibility of falling rock.

Westdahl Point offers very accessible specimens of interstadial stumps. Just north of the point, stumps project from the bank above the high-water shelf. Some are 10-15' tall, some have fallen as erosion exposed their roots, and undoubtedly others exist within the gravel banks and have not been uncovered. These spruce stumps date from four or five millenniums ago, when the Little Ice Age covered a Glacier Bay which had previously been ice-free long enough to allow the growth of mature forests. Glacial ice sheared off these tree trunks while a covering of glacial till, which has since eroded, protected their roots and stumps.

There are remains and ruins of mining activity at Nunatak Cove. The location is shown on the topo map, but mud flats and alders must be overcome to reach the spot. You'll need a strong motivation to get there.

McBride Glacier, flowing from the east into Muir Inlet, lies in a mile-wide canyon scoured out between Van Horn and McConnell ridges. Glaciers never completed the widening of this canyon, for rocky projections jut from the north and south, reaching to within a few hundred yards of each other. These rocky points enclose the half-mile-wide lagoon into which McBride's snout calves icebergs. A very narrow channel cuts from this lagoon into Muir Inlet, slicing through layers of sediments which have accumulated on the inlet side of the two points. Tidal action in this narrow, shallow channel is quite noticeable. Bergs float back and forth as the tide ebbs and flows. Large bergs can become grounded in the channel, blocking the exit as other bergs jam against them. Exercise caution here because of ice, and tidal action.

Riggs Glacier flows into Muir Inlet from the north, at the point where the main inlet makes a near-90° turn to the west. A few years ago, Riggs and McBride glaciers joined flows along the north side of McConnell Ridge. Only a few jumbles of ice now remain in this wide gully. However, Riggs does split

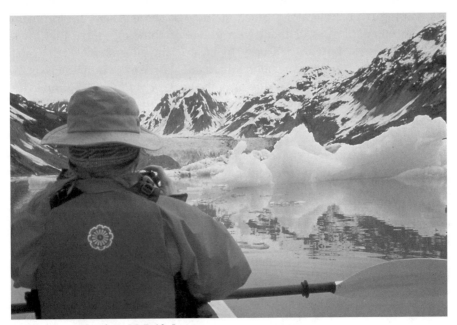

Laurie takes a shot from McBride Lagoon

its flow around a ridge lying due east of the snout, and around another, narrower ridge exposed in the snout itself near its north edge.

The lagoon at Riggs' snout only connects with the inlet at high tide. A gravel moraine intercedes at low water, and it is usually studded with bergs stranded there when the tide ebbed. Large waves can wash over this moraine on occasion when sizable bergs calve into the small lagoon, displacing huge volumes of water. Besides the views of various Riggs Glacier flows, you'll have a panoramic vista up the western end of Muir Inlet, a landscape locked in the ice age less than forty years ago. No kayakers floated here, enthralled by the sight of Riggs Glacier in 1960, as the inlet lay under hundreds of feet of ice.

Trip Description

This trip can be paddled as a continuation of Trip 3, by turning north at Point George as you leave Adams Inlet. By doing so, you will join the Trip 4 route at Point George. Otherwise, start Trip 4 at the Mt. Wright drop-off point (Map 3). From the drop-off, paddle north as described in Chapter 7 to Point George, on the north side of the Adams Inlet mouth.

From Point George (4 miles from the Mt. Wright drop-off) paddle north along the east shore of Muir Inlet. Any opposing current is generally weaker along shore, and you will have many small coves for protection if it is windy. Maquina Cove is 0.5 mile north of Point George. Another small but deeper cove is 0.5 mile farther. Both have landing beaches and possible campsites.

North of the second cove, the shoreline becomes steep for 1.5 miles, and rocky cliffs rise up nearly 1000 feet to form the Klotz Hills. Just past the point with the topo survey mark CUSH, you enter a shallow bay formed by the rounded inflow fan draining slopes cradling Casement Glacier. During clear weather there is a good view of the glacier here. Now, conifer forests begin thinning to patches on the shore and in the rising hills behind. Just past the Casement Glacier inflow fan, where the shoreline runs straight north, there is good camping on various old gravel benches that are not yet completely covered by alders (Map 5). Although the beach is made up of cobbles, landing can be accomplished (8 miles from the Mt. Wright drop-off).

There is a small bay at the south end of the Forest Creek inflow fan. Forest Creek is another melt stream from Casement Glacier, and its braided flows have created a mile-wide fan. Which of the fan's myriad channels flows, changes from time to time. Once past the Forest Creek fan, paddle 2 miles north northwest to Goose Cove. The relatively flat shore inland along this section allows an unobstructed view 4 miles northeast of 3580'-high Red Mountain. Goose Cove is small but quite deep, offering good wind protection and fine campsites. A minor stream enters the inlet just south of the cove.

Paddle out of Goose Cove, round the protecting point, and head north through the narrow channel that separates Sealers Island from the mainland.

Sealers Island is worth examining. Trees are definitely limited, but there is undergrowth on this low, rocky islet. Submerged rocks dot the channel between the island and the mainland. Continue 1 mile north from Sealers Island along a gravel beach that offers landing and camping possibilities; then enter Nunatak Cove (Map 5). Don't expect unlimited camping here, as much of the cove reverts to mud flats at low water. Good camping can be found on the cove's south shore on cobble or shingle beach.

As you leave Nunatak Cove heading north, a series of delightful beaches, in a 3-mile-long crescent, just beg to be explored. Campsites abound along this reach, and several streams enter the inlet. The low shore makes it possible to see inland, where eroding moraines with their sharply angled, top-plateaus contrast dramatically with the usual curved, glaciated landforms. The observant paddler will note how rapidly these moraines are being eroded.

At the north end of this crescent is a distinct cove, formed by the southern-most of two points making up the broad end of Van Horn Ridge (Map 6). Between the points, a tiny, angular cove invites exploring if you can delay your first encounter with a tidewater glacier for a few moments. Rounding the two points, you reach the broad tidal flats flanking the pincers-like entrance to McBride Glacier (15 miles from the Mt. Wright drop-off). The glacier itself comes into view abruptly, because of the narrow slot between the pincers. Across the lagoon the glacier snout presents a vertical, calving face reaching 75 feet or more in height.

At flood tide it is relatively easy to negotiate the channel into McBride Lagoon, but keep in mind that flood tides tend to concentrate the icebergs. If the ice is too thick to suit you, wait until ebb tide, when the bergs begin to flow outward from the lagoon through the channel, hopefully leaving you space to paddle in. As the water level drops, the bergs become more widely spaced. Always keep a watchful eye out when paddling among bergs.

Harbor seals use ice floes for resting, and pupping, in McBride Lagoon. Do not approach the pinnipeds, because they leave the ice when alarmed, and mother and offspring can become separated. Also, even if the berg density seems to permit it, do not approach any glacier face closer than the one-quarter-mile safety margin suggested by the Park Service. If you wish to camp near McBride Glacier, there are good sites just south around the point, as well as on a gravel beach 0.5 mile north of the McBride channel entrance.

Paddle 3 miles north from McBride Glacier along a mostly bare, rocky shore, with few haul-out spots. Shortly before you round the point at this shoreline's north end, Riggs Glacier comes into view, because it flows mainly from the north. Riggs displays an even more dramatic face than does McBride. A low gravel moraine, behind which Riggs calves into a small lagoon, presents a compelling landing spot (18 miles from the Mt. Wright drop-off). Walk across this gravel to get closer to the glacier face. Towering columns of white ice greet you, that are invariably undercut at the lagoon waterline. Caves and fissures extending into the ice reveal an incredible, deep blue color.

Exercise caution here. It is easy to feel secure simply because you are several hundred feet from the glacier's face, walking on smooth gravel, and safe from falling ice. It is not falling ice which could directly cause injury here; rather it's large waves arising in the lagoon should a large berg calve while you are there. The water level in the lagoon varies with the tide, and at high tide much of the gravel moraine is under water.

The end of this moraine, above the high-tide mark, provides one of those absolutely thrilling campsites. You can pitch your tent with a view of the glacier face a few hundred yards away. For years this was a drop-off point for kayakers, before awareness of its fragility became an issue. Overuse prompted the Park Service to discontinue stopping here, and move the drop-off first to Sebree Island and then to Mt. Wright. Recovery from overuse is slow at this latitude, but if this spot is used with loving care by paddlers, it can continue to offer a very special experience. From Riggs Glacier, it is possible to see nearly 5 miles west, toward the head of Muir Inlet. This moonscape, especially along the north shore, gives the spot an ethereal atmosphere.

You can return to the Mt. Wright pickup point from Riggs Glacier along the same east shore. Without detours, it is approximately 17 miles to your haul-out. Many paddlers, however, will want to return along Muir Inlet's west shore even though there are fewer campsites and fewer sheltering coves. From a distance, the 1000'-high cliffs of White Thunder Ridge do not appear very imposing. Paddling along

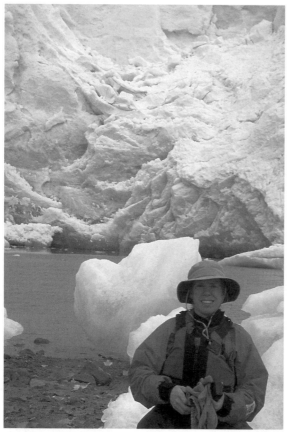

Laurie at Riggs Glacier   the base of these cliffs is

an entirely different matter. Be forewarned that there are no sheltering coves or landing sites for 4 miles along this shoreline. While it may be possible to haul out precariously on a talus slope, doing so is dangerous because of falling rocks.

A good camping area exists at the north end of the beach in the cove formed by Wolf Point. Tide flats at this beach's south end make it undesirable. There are also campsites near the north end of Stump Cove. The next decent camping opportunities south of Stump Cove are on Rowlee Point, on the south shore of the Wachusett Inlet mouth. Additional camping is available in Hunter Cove 1.5 miles south of Rowlee Point. If you search for a spot, you can find camping just south of the two points with the topo survey marks DENSON and MORSE, the latter just across Muir Inlet from Point George.

2.5 miles south of MORSE is the survey mark BULL, at the narrowest part of lower Muir Inlet. This is a good place to cross over to Muir Point, an open-water paddle of 1.5 miles. Then paddle south along the shore to the Mt. Wright pickup (34 miles round trip).

—•—🙐◊🙐—•—

We exited Adams Inlet, rounded Point George, and turned north into Muir Inlet. Our excitement was building. We had come to Glacier Bay to paddle among bergs and floes; now we were getting close to the tidewater glaciers. It was only partly our imagination that the air was beginning to take on a chill. Peaks to the east were mantled in deep snow, and we could see what appeared to be the edge of a cradled icefield.

Our progress northward was slowed by an ebb tide, and then it began to rain. Far to the west, a hole appeared in the clouds, and a distant area of the park was treated to glowing orange rays, gilding the edge of clouds as the sun dipped low. We settled for the night on an open, gravel-and-sand beach, near where a shed moose antler reposed in the moss, its tines bleached to a pearl grey. Moose tracks pockmarked the sand.

In the morning, we paddled north up Muir Inlet under a windless cloud cover. Within half an hour the sun burst through, turning the inlet to sparkling turquoise. Ashore, the light moss green of alders and cottonwoods contrasted with the dark spruce forest. Snowcaps shimmered. Even the harbor seals lingered before diving, seemingly reluctant to leave the brilliant surface world. The hospitable shore offered more camping spots than anyone could wish. The spruce forest diminished to occasional stands, the trees now small and immature. Alder and cottonwood were small and tenuous. Near Goose Cove we were treated to a brief glimpse west up the first 7 miles of Wachusett Inlet.

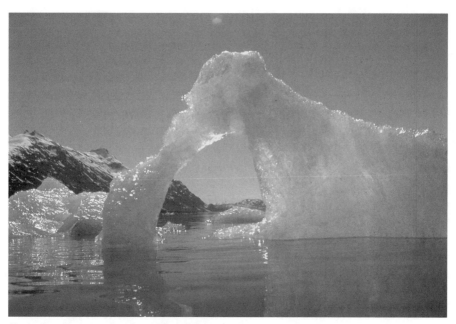

Bergs float in procession down Muir Inlet

Muir Inlet was narrowing, and at the same time growing starker. Along the west shore, arrow-straight White Thunder Ridge formed 1000'-high cliffs dropping vertically into the water. The first icebergs appeared ahead as shiny, white blinks on the surface. Then we could see that some were bluish, and others carried gravel and mud patches. Soon we passed near our first berg, and were fascinated by the myriad shapes of its projections. Then bergs were all around us, from shoebox size to half as big as a bus.

A hundred or more surf scoters, large black ducks with orange bills and white nape blazes paddled away from us, and then took wing. The birds made an impression, but then our eyes were drawn back to the unlimited shapes presented by dozens of sculptured bergs. Some had several holes melted through thin portions that projected skyward. Others looked polished, melted smooth with rounded contours. A few had jagged edges, newcomers to the frozen fleet held captive in the inlet by ebbing-and-flowing tides. We paddled on, carefully avoiding collisions with bergs. Tiny ice shards, nearly invisible on the surface, would clink occasionally along our hull like icecubes tinkling in a glass. Now the bergs were getting thicker.

We rounded the 0.5-mile-wide point capping Van Horn Ridge, and McBride Glacier sparkled there in the sun, a wide ribbon of white ice serrated across its breadth by fissures and cracks. Tide flats extended on either side of a narrow channel studded with grounded bergs. From a distance, the lagoon under McBride's snout seemed completely packed with ice. Bergs floated out to the inlet through the narrow channel like white ducks walking in a row, bobbing and turning in the ebbing current.

We carefully picked our way against the flow, dodging bergs moving like parade floats. A single iceberg, deep blue in the sunlight, and twice the others' height, dominated the center of the lagoon. Working carefully across a surface—half water, half ice—we moved closer to the snout. Occasional, sharp cracks and booms from the glacier gave the setting a strange, unearthly ambiance. Ice chunks fell from the vertical snout into the lagoon at intervals. As bergs collided their crunches and clinks added to the aura. Having come a long way to see this, to feel this, and to be in the middle of this, we were ecstatic because here we were.

Gone now was the warm air which had bathed us as we paddled up Muir Inlet. Here, cold air flowed constantly down the glacier face and spread out across the surface of McBride Lagoon. This wind made more unpredictable the dance of the icebergs waiting for the ebb flow to take them out through the channel and into Muir Inlet. Whether our perception or reality, the ice seemed to be closing in. After waiting longer than we felt comfortable, we turned the kayak and carefully joined the procession into Muir Inlet.

Later that day, we would repeat the glacial "close encounter" at Riggs Glacier. Each glacier had a different personality, a different look, and a different feel. Both were awe-inspiring. This was what we had come to Glacier Bay to see.

Chapter 9

TRIP 5 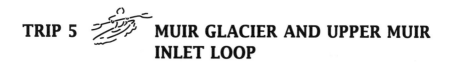 MUIR GLACIER AND UPPER MUIR INLET LOOP

Trip Details

Distance:	47 miles RT from Mt. Wright drop-off
	39 miles RT from Point George
	13 miles RT from Riggs Glacier
Time:	6-8 days (2 days from Riggs Glacier)
Rating:	Easy to Moderate
Maps:	NOAA Chart 17318; USGS Topos: Mt. Fairweather (D-1); Skagway (A-3) & (A-4)

Summary and Highlights

The main objective of this trip is to view Muir Glacier, once the most famous and frequently visited glacier on this continent. At the same time, you experience paddling along stark and unvegetated shores that are newly uncovered from the ice age. Your primary hazard is the cold water, measured at 40° Fahrenheit in May.

Area Features, Background, and Tips

As recently as 1960, glacial ice covered upper Muir Inlet northwest of a line between the north end of White Thunder Ridge and the west end of McConnell Ridge. This relative newness, more than any other factor, makes the upper inlet so stark and raw. Plant and animal life is just beginning here—once again.

Just west of the north end of White Thunder Ridge, is a gully beginning at the 1500' elevation, which now cradles a 3-mile long, unnamed remnant of Muir Glacier. West of this remnant, at 3000 feet, is Minnesota Ridge, bordering Burroughs Glacier. The sections of this ridge system visible from the water are the White Thunder Ridge ramparts towering above the inlet's west shore, and farther west in the inlet, the steep northern face of a 4000' ridge. They are impressive.

Most of the vegetation in upper Muir Inlet exists on the north-facing slope of the south shore. There has not been time for conifers to take hold; sizable trees here are mostly alder, with occasional small cottonwoods. The north-facing slope's heavier precipitation may have enabled this more rapid colonizing. Across the inlet on the north shore, alder colonization is almost nonexistent, and bare rock and gravels are pervasive.

There are numerous mountain goats on the north shore, indicating that there is sufficient plant life to sustain them, at least seasonally. The rodent population is sparse, but evidenced by the presence of raptors which subsist on them. Aside from the goats, other sizable land mammals are extremely scarce, or absent. Since land predators are not a problem, and indeed may be completely absent in the upper inlet, various sea birds nest on the mainland shore. Such rookeries are usually found on islands, where there is no predation from land animals.

Many animals have yet to arrive here, because Muir Glacier has beat a hasty retreat. Between 1972 and 1982, receding ice uncovered more than 3 miles of inlet, freeing new land. The rapid melting and disintegration of the glacier resulted in an inlet clogged with bergs and debris. It was impossible to approach close enough to see the glacier's face at various times in the past.

When John Muir visited in 1880 and 1890, the glacier, that was to bear his name, filled the inlet to Muir Point. From his accounts, the ice melt at that time was relatively slow. For decades in the early 1900s, cruise-ship visits to Muir Glacier were popular and the glacier enjoyed worldwide fame. Then, periods of rapid melt clogged the inlet with ice, and cruise ships could not reach the face; they visited other glaciers to offer passengers the spectacle of calving icebergs. Today, Muir Glacier is grounded, and does not calve bergs directly into tidewater. A period of advancing ice can begin again for Muir Glacier at any time. Or, the face may remain grounded where it is for decades, or even continue to recede. Glaciers do not react to current climatic changes, and are impossible to predict. Of the nine or more tidewater glaciers in Glacier Bay, several are advancing, some are retreating, and others remain static.

Particularly in upper Muir Inlet, the water often becomes "banded," where streams of fresh water entering the inlet float on top of the denser salt water. Bands often have individual colors, caused by the varying sedimentary load of the fresh water. Several sizable runoff streams pour into Muir Inlet. The results are bands of varicolored water that can stretch for miles along the inlet, until they are finally diffused by tidal currents.

Camping in upper Muir Inlet is very limited. Many paddlers have camped at Riggs Glacier, and made the very long day trip to Muir Glacier and back. Doing so severely limits the amount of time that can be spent at Muir Glacier, or floating and taking in the sights on the upper inlet. The 13-mile round trip may also be difficult for some paddlers. With a little searching, minimal camp-sites can be found. Limited camping is possible beside a meltwater stream that flows down the south shore 1.5 miles west of the north point of White Thunder Ridge. But this is still a considerable distance from Muir Glacier.

A few small streams have created sedimentary deposits along the north shore where camping is possible. First find a landing beach, and then search for a spot flat and large enough to pitch a tent. While some of these sites may be very tight for space, there are often other rewards such as views, birdlife, and, of course, solitude. Winter storms can create suitable camping beaches in small coves or, just as easily, wash them away. Drainage streams, swollen with snowmelt or rain, can throw up flat gravel benches, or remove those previously deposited. So such campsites are, seasonally, where you find them.

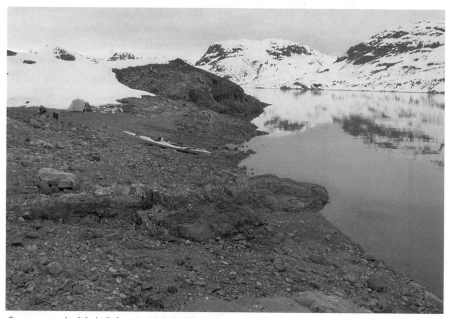

Snug camp in Muir Inlet near Muir Glacier

One such site is located 136° 17′ west longitude, near several small points on the north shore of the inlet. It's also possible to camp near the face of Muir Glacier, on its west side. This inflow wash area is constantly changing, so make sure that any site selected is well above high water, and secure from other hazards associated with rock and ice.

Trip Description

Since the drop-off point serving Muir Inlet is at Mt. Wright, paddlers have to travel over part of the route described in Chapter 7 (Trip 3) and all of the route described in Chapter 8 (Trip 4) before reaching the beginning point for Trip 5. The upper Muir Inlet and Muir Glacier paddle is an extension of the tour of McBride and Riggs glaciers. If glaciers are your goal and time is short, you can bypass Adams Inlet travelling northbound, and plan to visit there on your return if time allows.

This trip begins at Riggs Glacier, 17 miles north of the Mt. Wright drop-off point (Map 6). Put the fascinating ice face of Riggs to your stern, and begin by paddling west along the north shore of upper Muir Inlet. Watch for mountain goats here; they are especially easy to spot against the bare slopes of the north shore. Across the inlet, imposing cliffs forming the north end of White Thunder Ridge are 1.5 miles away. Notice how your sense of distance is distorted by the ridge's towering rock face. Follow the north shore unless you need a place to camp.

Keeping a lookout for goats close to the water, paddle west along a straight, 2-mile segment of the north shore. Don't be surprised if the shoreline doesn't match the one shown on NOAA chart #17318, for this is a very new inlet, and gravel outflows can fill in coves, or create outwash fans in a matter of months. Note the array of small points on your right at the end of the straight section. Limited campsites can usually be found here. During early season, inflow streams also provide drinking water. Camping

Rocky Mountain Goat peers down from his moraine

possibilities on the south shore along this section are practically nonexistent. The irregular shoreline extends to a point 3 miles west of Riggs Glacier. Here Muir Inlet bends 45° to the north.

Muir Inlet bends again—this time directly north—2.5 miles beyond the first bend. Soon, you get your first view of the face of Muir Glacier, although it is still nearly a mile and a half away. Both shores of the inlet are extremely steep at this point. The shore on your right consists of low-to-medium cliffs, while the left (west) shore is the steep side of a 4000′ unnamed peak. The south and west shore has supported alder growth along the section just passed, but now both shorelines exhibit equal, inhospitable starkness.

The best landing spots at Muir Glacier (6.5 miles from Riggs Glacier) depending upon the tide, are found near the glacier's outflow stream. A very sticky mud is present here, but by walking on the more gravelly spots, or in the stream itself, you can avoid most of the mud. It's only a short walk on the gravel moraine to the ice face. Ice does fall from the Muir snout, so do not get too close. Paddlers can often find a minimal campsite a short distance from the west side of the glacier face. Your main consideration here is the hazards of falling rock or ice, and high tide. Keep in mind that glacial winds often blow near the Muir face. From this point, retrace your route to Riggs Glacier, possibly following the opposite shore for a different perspective of the upper inlet. Riggs Glacier is 6.5 miles away.

⊷ ⊷ ⊨⬦⊨ ⊷ ⊷

Two mountain goats, just yards from the shoreline and a few feet from Riggs Glacier, munched hungrily on sparse plants that were invisible to us. What had they found to eat here? Voicing that thought reminded us that it was long past lunch time. We drifted and ate also, while watching the goats. In the still air Muir Inlet was glassy, reflecting the 1500′ cliffs where the inlet turns west around the north end of White Thunder Ridge. Turning west, we paddled along the north shore. A bald eagle flapped by, paying no attention to us. Minutes later, we noticed a northern harrier, flying its jerky, stop-and-go hunting pattern over a rocky knob. Apparently there were rodents there, competing for sparse vegetation with some goats now coming into view.

As we neared the end of the inlet the breeze picked up, a cold, gravity wind sliding off Muir Glacier and out onto the fiord. We rounded a point and headed northwest; a mile and a half later the inlet turned and headed due north. Now we could see the face of Muir Glacier, grounded at low tide behind a hundred yards of gravel beach.

The immense ice cave, walls the color of deep, blue sapphire, that reached far back under the glacier in the center of the snout, took our breath away. We landed, and finding nothing to secure the boat to, half dragged it out of the water. Cameras in hand, we picked our way along the melt stream, avoiding pools and steep gravel banks, to a spot near the cave opening. Fallen blocks of ice discouraged any thought of entering the cave, or even approaching closely. We stood, awestruck, for a time; then tried to capture the true perspective of the place on film. While we lingered, two small rockfalls reminded us that the surroundings were new, unstable land.

Finally, aware that the flooding tide was inching near our boat, we left. Now the glacial wind was at our back, moving us swiftly south and east, away from Muir Glacier. Our last view of the face, from a different angle, revealed a nanny and kid browsing on the east slope, just a few hundred yards from the ice. Were they eating lichens? Or have more complex plant forms established here? Looking upward at the cliff while rounding the point, we noticed a single, green fern affixed tenuously to a rock in the middle of its dinner-plate-sized seep.

It had been a long day, one full of excitement and exhilaration. Suddenly we felt tired, ready to stop. Around a sharp point, a foot-wide stream flowed in at a beach just wide enough for our boat. Steep ridges on either side blocked the wind. We looked at each other; then headed the boat in. Several feet above the tide mark, the tiny stream had scoured a shelf and piled a small gravel bank just large enough for our tent. As it turned out, this spot was one of the finest campsites of our trip. We found shelter, there was a good spot for the boat, and 3 feet from the tent was a sparkling stream, singing a quiet melody. We set up camp, snacked a bit, and feeling renewed, looked more carefully at our surroundings.

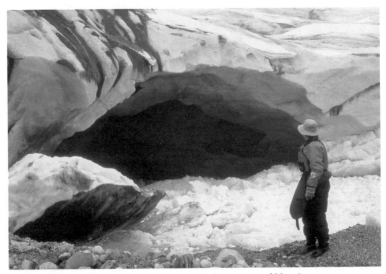

Snout of Muir Glacier presently features a huge cave of blue ice

Along the shore 30 yards away, two black oystercatchers were performing a courtship ritual. Another pair stood together on a rock a short distance away, looking territorial. A glaucous-winged gull, perched on a high knoll, made us aware that three varieties of gulls, paired for nesting, occupied territories surrounding our campsite. Luckily, our chosen site had not disturbed the birds.

In the lengthy evening twilight, we sat for a long time looking out of the tent. The birds around us had quieted, the wind dropped, and Muir Inlet became glassy. We could feel the newness. In this rapidly birthing place we were privileged spectators. At 10:00 P.M., with broad daylight just beginning to change to summer's half-dark, we crawled into our sleeping bags.

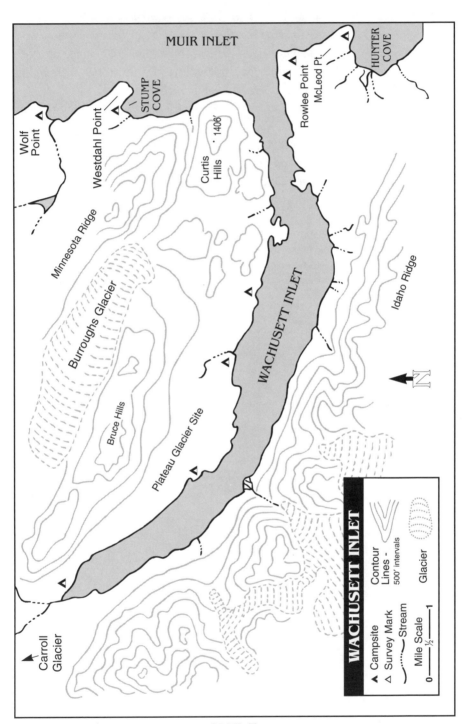

MUIR INLET

MAP 7

Chapter 10

TRIP 6 WACHUSETT INLET LOOP

Trip Details

Distance: 20 miles RT from inlet mouth

Time: 2-3 days

Rating: Easy

Map: NOAA Chart 17318; USGS topos: Mt. Fairweather (D-1) & (D-2)

Summary and Highlights

Trip 6 may be done in conjunction with Trips 3, 4, and 5. Rapidly eroding landforms and hanging glaciers are the major features of Wachusett Inlet. Moraines left by Burroughs and Plateau glaciers are undergoing rapid erosion, resulting in expanding gullies and canyons. Land surfaces along much of the north shore of Wachusett Inlet are being constantly rearranged. The resultant alluvium fills coves and bays along the inlet's shoreline, changing its contours. On the south shore, Idaho Ridge, with its attendant glacier remnants and ice fields, projects skyward to more then 5000 feet. These impressive snowcaps provide the backdrop for a paddle in Wachusett Inlet. The main hazards in the inlet are the cold water, and the possibility of sudden wind and waves.

Area Features, Background, and Tips

Viewed on the chart, Wachusett Inlet looks like the bottom claw of giant pincers formed by the two western arms of Muir Inlet. The 12-mile-long arc of Wachusett curves west and then northwest, between Idaho Ridge to the south, and Bruce Hills to the north. Just northeast of Bruce Hills, Burroughs Glacier lies cradled between them and Minnesota Ridge. Both Burroughs

Glacier and Cushing Glacier, farther northwest, previously entered Wachusett Inlet alongside Carroll Glacier. They have now both receded several miles to the north and east. Along the northeast shore of Wachusett Inlet, in a depression you can't see this side of Bruce Hills, is the former site of Plateau Glacier, once instrumental in forming of the inlet. Only the lower one-third of Wachusett Inlet was free of ice in 1950. By 1966, only the upper third was locked in the ice age. Today, alder, willows, and cottonwoods are establishing rapidly, especially in the lower reaches of the inlet.

The north shore of the upper inlet provides some graphic lessons in erosion. Moraines left here by Burroughs and Plateau glaciers are prominent. The rapid wearing away of these features by water erosion is just as unmistakable. The sloughing banks, and the recent, jagged canyons and gullies, all indicate that flowing water is leveling this landscape. This rapid erosion of newly uncovered moraines and other topographic features is undoubtedly responsible for the ever-changing shoreline. Your marine chart will be fine for depicting the overall shape of Wachusett Inlet, but don't count on it for accuracy when it comes to details such as small coves or bays. These features are filled so rapidly with wash-out gravel that the chart has little value for identifying such spots.

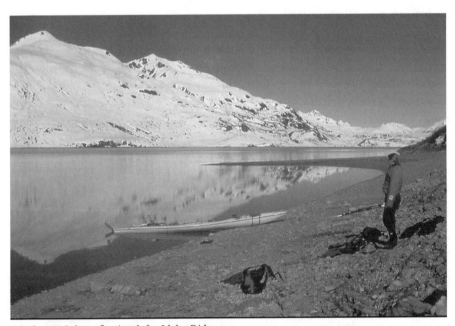

Wachusett Inlet reflecting lofty Idaho Ridge

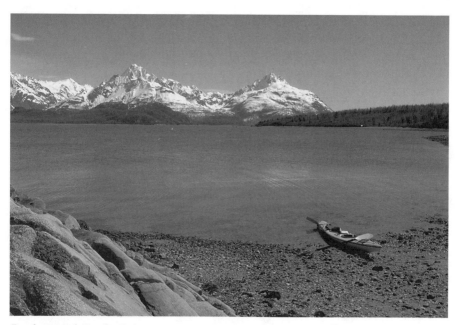

Beach at south Rowlee Point

A memorable feature of Wachusett Inlet is the intimate presence of Idaho Ridge rising steeply along the south shore, and the sometimes visible peaks projecting above it, to the west. Studded with dozens of glacier and icefield remnants, this snowy world caps the peninsula between Wachusett and the west arm of Glacier Bay, 6 miles away. Tidal flats in this inlet are often deeply scored and furrowed by floating ice where tides and winds have pushed bergs across the mud and gravel bottom. Look for these signs on exposed tide flats along the inlet.

The same forces rapidly altering the landscape through erosion are also creating new camping possibilities. Look for excellent campsites on both sides of Rowlee Point, at the inlet mouth. Heading up the inlet, the next feasible camping area is 3.5 miles away on the north shore, beyond a small, rocky peninsula. There are good sites for the next mile or more along this shore. Look for camping spots by exploring near the small, rocky points which jut from shore. At the end of the inlet, 2 points jut from the east and west shores near latitude 59°. Beyond these points, camping is unwise because of mud flats.

Unfortunately, all that can be seen of Carroll Glacier from near the inlet's head is a number of moraines resembling huge, rounded piles of gravel stretching across the valley. The glacier itself has withdrawn some distance to the west, and is not visible. Wachusett Inlet creates its own mini-climate, which differs somewhat from other inlets because fog often forms in the upper reaches. Winter snows remain along the shoreline longer than in other inlets, often not melting until June.

Trip Description

The beginning point for Trip 6, Wachusett Inlet, is at the middle of Trip 4, about halfway between Adams Inlet and McBride Glacier (Map 5). Because Wachusett is unlikely to be a sole destination, and is more often visited in conjunction with other locations in Muir Inlet, its description and mileage begin at the mouth of Wachusett Inlet.

From Muir Inlet, paddle due west into the mouth of Wachusett Inlet (Map 7). There are good campsites on both sides of Rowlee Point, although there is no potable water. Soon the inlet mouth narrows to less than half a mile. Paddle along either shore, as both are interesting. Along the north shore 1 mile from the entrance, mussels carpet the intertidal area, which looks like a bright, purplish-blue band at low tide. Across the way, near the south shore, are submerged rocks.

On the south shore, 1 mile farther, is a rounded peninsula. Paddling 0.5 mile west from the rounded peninsula, on the opposite north shore, you'll find a tidal flat extending behind a craggy, rocky peninsula which may become an island during very high tides. West of this point the inlet begins to widen, and curve gently northward.

Most paddlers will want to follow the north shore west of the craggy peninsula, partly because the wind is slightly less here, but mostly because of the spectacular view of Idaho Ridge across the inlet. Charts show an inflowing stream and a tiny, inland estuary behind the rounded, north-shore peninsula. Although they may still exist during the highest of tides, you'll need good luck to find them. Good camping can be found at several sites in this general area. The inlet bends again to the north 3 miles west of the peninsula, around a very broad point (6 miles from Muir Inlet). Near this point, high on the west side of a 3500' peak, two glacier tongues flow down from either side. Melt streams from them tumble and fall down the steep slope into tidewater.

The imposing mounds and ridges to the north here are the Bruce Hills, which were mostly deposited and shaped by Burroughs Glacier. Interestingly, at this time Burroughs was moving northwest, while its companion Carroll Glacier, which joined to form Wachusett Inlet, flowed in the opposite direction. Mile-wide Wachusett Inlet extends northwest for another 4 miles, where it narrows between opposing rock points. Alluvium clogs the inlet there, forming extensive tidal flats. Good campsites can be found southeast of these rocky points. Here, at 59° latitude, it is 10 miles back to Muir Inlet.

Small bergs were floating out as we rounded Curtis Hills and paddled west into Wachusett Inlet. Within a short distance our surroundings changed. In Muir Inlet the winter snowpack had melted to an elevation hundreds of feet above tidewater. But here, in Wachusett in mid-May, 3 feet of snow carpeted the landscape right down to the tide line. A closer look at the bergs floating sedately down the inlet showed that they were flat sheets, actually part of the snow layer that blanketed much of the shore.

Wachusett was setting the mood around us as we paddled. The sun gave up poking holes through the scudding clouds, and the afternoon light turned a somber gray. Although we had been looking for a campsite for more than an hour, the snow obscured any likely stopping place. Finally we landed on a sloping beach of mud and gravel. At the high-water mark, a 3' bank marked the beginning of a snowfield of the same thickness. Despairing of finding a ready-made site for our tent, I began stomping out a compacted platform in the snow large enough to accommodate our camp. After falling through the snow several times, I had to move and pack more snow to make a patchwork surface.

Uncertain about anchoring the tent and tieing the boat, Laurie wasn't thrilled to spend the night on the snowpack. Her exploring farther along the beach revealed a niche at the base of a near-vertical rock bank that we judged to be 3 feet above high water. We quickly abandoned the snow camp in favor of making a level platform from loose scree just shy of our tent size, but close enough. Before we finished eating, a steady rain began to fall.

A subconscious prompting awakened me at night with the urge to check the tide level. Raindrops were silver streaks across the flashlight beam, which revealed still, black water a few feet below our tent. Satisfied that we were safe and the boat was secure, I pulled the sleeping bag around me and soon rain drumming on the tent sent me back to dreamland.

Brilliant, early-morning sunlight flooded the inlet when we got up, glaring off the snow and making us don sunglasses even before the rays reached our camp. In the still air, Wachusett turned into a giant reflection pond. The far shore, which had been cloud-shrouded the day before, sloped abruptly to a ridge line far above and was snow-mantled down to the waterline. Capping the ridge at intervals, and creeping down gullies were glacier remnants, with their characteristic, scale-like surfaces partially disguised under last winter's snow. Glaciers and a jagged ridgetop danced on the water in front of us; it was a Wachusett welcome to remember.

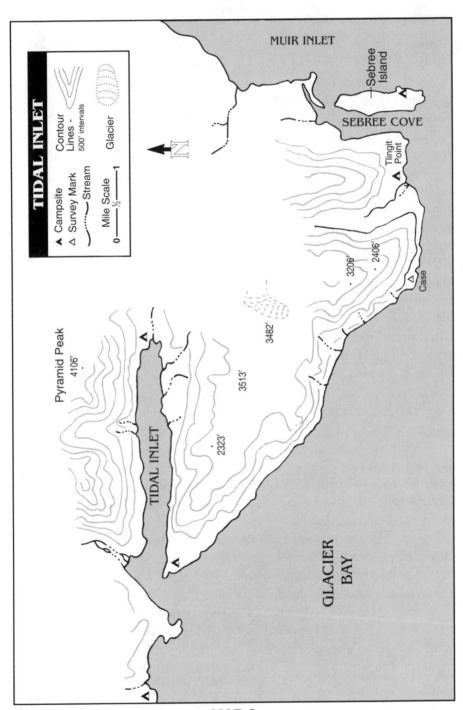

MAP 8

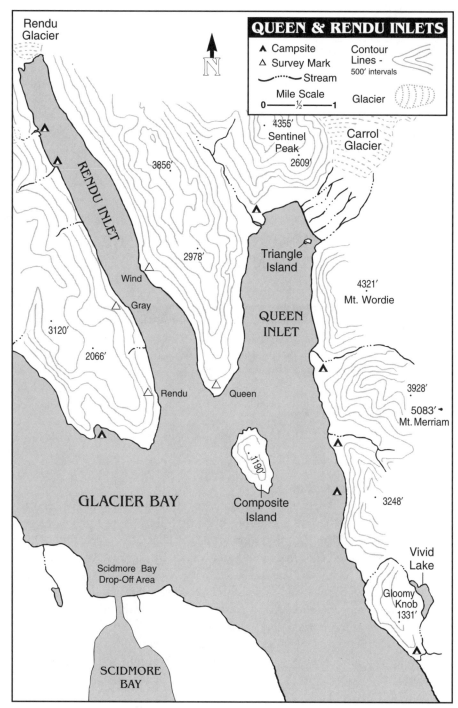

Rendu
Glacier

QUEEN & RENDU INLETS

▲ Campsite
△ Survey Mark
Stream

Mile Scale
0 —— ½ —— 1

Contour
Lines -
500′ intervals

Glacier

4355′
Sentinel
Peak
2609′

Carrol
Glacier

3856′

RENDU INLET

2978′

Triangle
Island

4321′
Mt. Wordie

QUEEN
INLET

Wind

Gray

3120′

2066′

Rendu

Queen

3928′

5083′
Mt. Merriam

GLACIER BAY

1190′

Composite
Island

3248′

Vivid
Lake

Gloomy
Knob
1331′

Scidmore Bay
Drop-Off Area

SCIDMORE
BAY

MAP 9

Chapter 11

TRIP 7 TIDAL, QUEEN, AND RENDU INLETS
FROM MT. WRIGHT

Trip Details

Distance:	80 miles RT from Mt. Wright drop-off
	60 miles from Mt. Wright drop-off to Scidmore Bay pickup.
	70 miles RT from Scidmore Bay drop-off
Time:	6-10 days
Rating:	Moderate to Difficult
Maps:	NOAA Chart 17318; USGS Topos: Mt. Fairweather (D-1), (D-2) & (D-3); Skagway (A-5)

Summary and Highlights

This trip exposes you to the open-water conditions of Glacier Bay. Shortly after your drop-off there is a crossing of Muir Inlet. A few miles later you begin paddling upwind (usually) along miles of Glacier Bay coastline which provide few sheltered sites from wind and waves. By contrast, the three inlets to be visited are calm and serene, each with a distinct personality you'll remember. The waterfalls, and other sights you'll see, your feeling of solitude a pristine landscape engenders, and your own rich reflections; these will form the basis for your memories. Rendu Inlet is designated non-motorized water from May 1 to September 15. Camping is good at many locations within the inlets, and at a few other places along the way. You will see marbled murrelets, murres, and cormorants, birds which favor the larger, open-water environment of the main bay.

Cold water is once again a hazard here, especially in areas where strong winds can bring on sudden waves. Winds can arise while you are between sheltered shoreline features, or in the middle of a crossing. Carefully assess your skills and experience; you must be capable of reaching a shelter should such conditions arise. This trip involves crossing Muir Inlet, an optional 1-mile crossing to Composite Island, and ends with a 2-mile crossing of Glacier Bay.

Area Features, Background, and Tips

Tidal Inlet is a 4-mile-long waterway that never exceeds 0.5 mile in width. The glacier responsible for this narrow fiord is long gone. It flowed west from a low saddle 3 miles east of the inlet head. The eastern flow of ice from

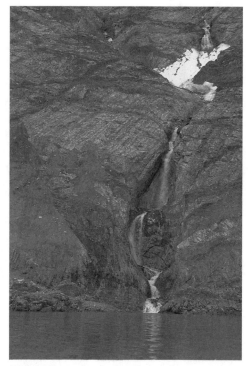

Waterfalls are frequent and varied in Rendu Inlet

this same saddle crept southeast through what is now Ice Valley into Muir Inlet just north of Sebree Island. Hundreds of feet above the water, on the north shore of Tidal Inlet, you can see clear signs of a giant landslide. It probably occurred in the 1860s, when the ice which supported the steep side walls melted. Alder is healing the gash slowly, but the scar is still plainly visible. The slope is precipitous enough that more sliding could occur at any time.

Queen Inlet, an 8-mile trip north, is sheltered behind Composite Island, a mile-long continuation of the ridge between Queen and Rendu inlets which thrusts its rounded, glaciated dome nearly 900 feet above the bay. Opposite Composite Island, on the east, mainland shore, is an alder-dotted, 0.5-mile-wide outwash fan. It's from a glacial stream running down the slopes of Mt. Merriam. Another glacial melt stream 2 miles north, which drains the watershed between Mt. Merriam and Mt. Wordie, flows into Queen Inlet. Aside from the beach at the inlet head, these two outwash fans offer the only camping possibilities in Queen Inlet.

Carroll Glacier can only be seen from the entrance to the inlet, near the north end of Composite Island. It has retreated 3 miles or more, leaving its melt stream to wend through very prominent, gravel moraines. This mile-wide outwash is a playing field for the capricious stream, which winds a braided course through a current selection of its myriad channels. Over the last 80 years, Carroll Glacier has alternately retreated or advanced on the gravel plains some distance inland from the inlet. Whether Carroll will advance to tidewater again in the near future, no one knows.

At 4355 feet, Sentinel Peak dominates the landscape north of Queen Inlet. A stream draining its western slopes has created a 0.5-mile-long outwash fan. With the exception of the gravel beach at the foot of Sentinel Peak, where campsites can be found, and the outwash fans, the shoreline of Queen Inlet is quite steep.

A narrow ridge separates Queen Inlet from Rendu Inlet. Rendu Glacier has had periods of advance as recently as the 1960s, when it was calving bergs into tidewater. It is now well grounded, and no bergs float the inlet except those which currents bring from other sources. Rendu is a 0.7-mile-wide, steep-sided fiord that offers rewarding views.

It is no exaggeration to call Rendu Inlet a world of waterfalls. Here, more than in any other Glacier Bay inlet, water spectacles streak both shorelines. It is not uncommon to count a dozen or more falls per mile of shoreline. Just when you think you have seen all possible variations, a new one comes along that either separates into braids, free falls for considerable distance, does a rhythmic cascade over rocky ledges, or a combination of all imaginable forms. Paddling Rendu is worth it for the waterfalls alone.

Trip Description

In keeping with the trip descriptions in this book, which together add up to a complete circumnavigation of Glacier Bay, the beginning point for this trip is at the Mt. Wright drop-off. **There is, however, another option: that of starting the trip at the Scidmore Bay drop-off.** Doing so reduces the total mileage, but involves an open-water, west-to-east crossing of Glacier Bay, and another crossing upon the return trip. If you start at Scidmore Bay, the route described here can be paddled in reverse.

From the Mt. Wright drop-off, paddle 2 miles north to the westernmost part of Muir Point (Map 3). Choosing calm weather, make the 1.5-mile crossing of Muir Inlet to the west shore. Turn south along the west shore, and paddle 1.5 miles to the shallow bay and tidal flats where the Ice Valley stream enters. Continue 1 mile south of the stream to Caroline Point. After rounding this point, head 0.5 mile southwest to Sebree Island, and then 1.5 miles south to the southern tip of Sebree (8 miles from the Mt. Wright drop-off).

There are camping sites on the east side of Sebree on either side of a small point 0.5 mile north of the south end of the island (Map 8). From the south tip of Sebree, paddle west, crossing the mouth of Sebree Cove. This cove is now largely an extensive mud flat. Continue past Tlingit Point, where your chart may show a small island just offshore. There are landing possibilities along the shore within the first 2 miles west of Tlingit Point, but beyond that, there are few sheltered sites for 3 miles. The shore is either steep cliffs or banks, or jumbles of talus dangerous to land upon. If landing really becomes necessary, look for small, distinct rocky points which have gravel beaches instead of talus along their south shores.

The shoreline clearly bends to the northwest 3 miles west of Sebree Island, at the topo survey mark CASE. Now you are in Glacier Bay proper, without shelter from northwesterly breezes. A very shallow, crescent-shaped indentation in the shore extends 2.5 miles northwest from CASE. Half a dozen short, cascading streams enter tidewater along this section. Feasible spots to land are few, and change in location as storms rearrange the small but sporadic gravel beaches each season.

From the north end of the crescent, paddle 3 miles northwest to the spit of land which defines the south entrance to Tidal Inlet. Just before reaching the inlet mouth, you'll find that this point forms a sizable crescent beach with a considerable grassy area above the tidal zone. There are good campsites on this beach, but no water is available (16 miles from the Mt. Wright drop-off).

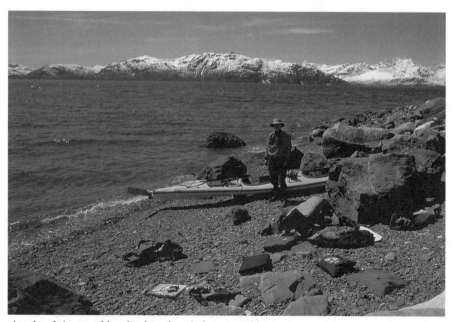

Any beach is a good beach when the wind starts to blow

From the point, turn east and paddle 4 miles to the head of Tidal Inlet. The only campsites deep inside are near the stream at the inlet head. As you leave the inlet, campsites can also be found near the stream on the north shore, which has built a small fan just opposite the south point. There are good campsites 1 mile farther west, on both sides of a small, 0.3-mile long hammerhead point.

Just inside a small but distinct limestone point 0.7 mile west of the hammerhead point are a series of fine gravel beaches, with excellent campsites well above high water. Here, bare, glaciated limestone slopes run upward forming rounded terraces, where mountain goats are often seen. Bears eat kinnikinik berries which grow seasonally on the terraces. A stream running in here originates 1 mile north in Vivid Lake, and drains a small but picturesque valley (Map 9). From the limestone point, paddle 2 miles northwest along the rounded, near-vertical cliffs of Gloomy Knob to another outlet stream—this one running northwest—from Vivid Lake. For 0.5 mile on both sides of the stream the shoreline is less precipitous.

Paddle 1 mile north of the stream, passing a rounded point. The shoreline curves north along this reach, as you approach the entrance to Queen Inlet at Composite Island. Continue 1 mile farther and you will be opposite the south end of Composite Island (29 miles from the Mt. Wright drop-off). This is the location of the Queen Inlet drop-off used prior to 1998. Paddle 2 miles north until you reach Queen Inlet's first, sizable inflow stream. Camping is possible at various sites along the 0.5-mile-wide outwash fan. Continue 2 miles north to where another stream has created a sizable fan. This stream, which has formed a bay north of the fan, drains the southwest slopes of Mt. Wordie. Several locations here are suitable for camping.

Steep cliffs of Mt. Wordie abut the shoreline for the next 2.5 miles. Then, you reach the tidal flats and gravel outwash of Carroll Glacier. Triangle Island, located here, may not be an island when you arrive, depending upon tide levels. Carroll's outwash gravels, and the mud flats guarding them, are a mile wide. Paddle past the outwash fan to the inlet head; then turn west and go 1 mile to a large outwash whose stream originates west of Sentinel Peak. This outwash fan provides the only suitable campsite in the upper inlet. From the Sentinel Peak stream, paddle 4 miles south along the steep, west shore of Queen Inlet to the point with the topo survey mark QUEEN (42 miles from the Mt. Wright drop-off). This is a good place from which to cross a channel of the bay and explore Composite Island. Since it is 1 mile to the island, and 3.5 miles to circumnavigate it, your total mileage for this side trip is 5.5 miles.

Rounding the promontory with the survey mark QUEEN, which separates Queen and Rendu inlets, head north into Rendu. The east shore curves northwest forming a shallow crescent for 2.5 miles, to a point with the topo survey mark WIND. If necessary your camp can be made here above a tiny but protected gravel beach. By now you will have discovered that Rendu Inlet is known for waterfalls. The splashing, roaring, and singing of falls will serenade you along both shores of Rendu Inlet.

Continue 4 miles northwest from WIND to the head of Rendu Inlet. There are few camping possibilities here. Turn southeast, now following the west shore of the inlet, and within 1.5 miles you will come to a sizable stream entering from the west. This is the melt flow from Romer Glacier. Here you can find a campsite. Paddle 2 miles southeast passing two more streams which flow down the steep inlet sides. There are possible campsites by each of these. There is a small rocky point with the topo survey mark GRAY 1.5 miles beyond the second of the two streams. From GRAY paddle 2 miles south to the point with the survey mark RENDU. It is 1 mile south from RENDU to the point of the peninsula separating Rendu Inlet from Glacier Bay (56 miles from the Mt. Wright drop-off, not including the Composite Island side trip).

Should you wish to return to the Mt. Wright pickup from here, the distance is about 24 miles excluding inlet and cove exploration. Paddle cross-channel to Composite Island, then around its southern end, and then cross-channel again to the east shore. Retrace the trip route in this chapter to Mt. Wright. If your destination is the Scidmore Bay pickup or Trip 8 locales, paddle around the peninsula point 1 mile to a small, sheltered bay with a good campsite. (This bay is the starting point for Trip 8.) Leaving the bay, it is 2 miles across open water from the protecting point to the west shore of Glacier Bay. Pick calm conditions for the crossing. Once across, the Scidmore Bay north-entrance channel will probably be east of you. Make sure you check on the exact location of the pickup point before leaving park headquarters, as it is moved around depending upon salmon runs and brown bear activity.

━━━ ≣◆≣ ━━━

We were blessed by clear days and lots of sunshine, thanks to a high-pressure system that was then over Glacier Bay. The downside was the accompanying wind. We were looking forward to the calm of narrow, protected inlets after enduring headwinds and waves while paddling northwest up the coast from Muir Inlet. The protected gravel beach just south of the Tidal Inlet entrance provided many campsite choices, all gloriously free of wind. Our tent went up in a spot that did not intrude on the bald-eagle pair nesting in cottonwoods behind us, and well clear of the comical pair of black oystercatchers that tried to divert us away from their nest when we once walked too close. The next morning, we entered Tidal Inlet and a world of waterfalls. Some come sliding down cliffs, some cascade from bench to bench, and others hide in the vegetation until we view them head on. This is what we will remember about Tidal Inlet.

After 7 grueling miles paddling against a head wind, we enter Queen Inlet via the channel east of Composite Island. Ahead in Queen Inlet we can see glassy water. If the wind has changed, so has the shoreline. Gone are most of the spruce which sprinkled much of Tidal Inlet. Patches of struggling alders are the style here, bordering streams and scrabbling for toeholds wherever possible on the mountain sides.

High on our list of must-sees for Glacier Bay are humpback whales. Even knowing that our early season expedition here will likely be over before the whales complete their migration from the south, we spend lots of time searching for distant spouts. Maybe we'll be lucky and spot an early arrival. Just as we paddle onto the mirror surface east of Composite Island, that distinctive, sharp whoosh of a whale breathing sounds behind us. Turning the boat, we see two humpbacks, a cow and a calf, surface, blow, and slip back into the depths in one fluid motion. The humpbacks have arrived!

Today in Queen Inlet ours is a paddle over glass. We complete our exploration of the shoreline, but are still a little disappointed. Carroll Glacier, having receded far behind the giant moraines at the head of the inlet, has eluded us again. As we approach the end of the peninsula separating Queen and Rendu inlets, Composite Island hangs as if painted upon the glassy fiord.

Getting from Queen Inlet to Rendu requires only rounding a point. There are few indications of the steady breeze in the main channel by the point, but we can see whitecaps 3 miles south. We are content to turn north into Rendu Inlet. Here, as in Tidal Inlet, our senses are assailed by waterfalls. We could pick almost any

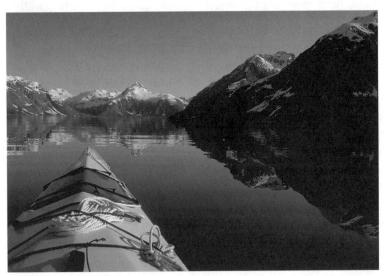

Paddling up Queen Inlet

size, and whether we preferred a direct plunge into tidewater, a bounce off an intervening shelf, or a series of cascades; there was never any disappointment. Some falls appear unheralded by a visible stream above, fall for a short distance, and then disappear again into a rock jumble. Others braid into misty ropes for a ways, then rejoin in one flow to continue the ballet to tidewater. Both shores compete in this waterfall extravaganza.

Rendu Glacier—though grounded—remains within sight. The view is a fitting finale to our visit to these three, mild-mannered inlets. Turning south again, we can see 8 miles to the west shore of Composite Island, the rest hidden behind the intervening point. The steep shorelines between us and the point are faithfully reflected on the still surface, distorted only by our bow wave. We are in no hurry. The boat moves easily, but slowly, responding to our reluctance to leave the magic of this sheltering trio of inlets.

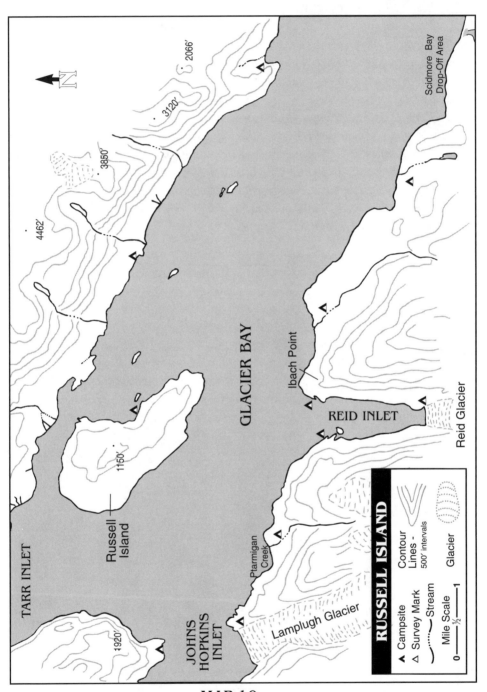

RUSSELL ISLAND

GLACIER BAY

TARR INLET

JOHNS
HOPKINS
INLET

REID INLET

Ibach Point

Reid Glacier

Scidmore Bay
Drop-Off Area

Russell
Island

1150'

1920'

4462'

3850'

3120'

2066'

Ptarmigan
Creek

Lamplugh Glacier

N

▲ Campsite

△ Survey Mark

Contour
Lines -
500' intervals

⌄
⌄
⌄

Stream

Glacier

Mile Scale

0   ½   1

MAP 10

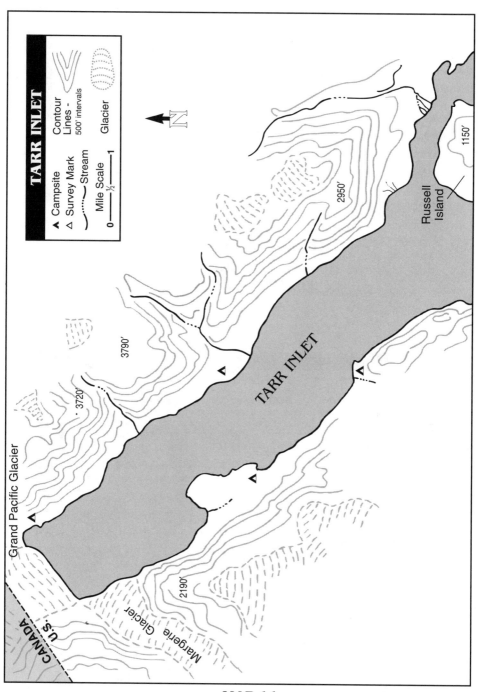

TARR INLET

▲ Campsite
△ Survey Mark

Contour
Lines -
500' intervals

⋯⋯ Stream

Glacier

Mile Scale
0 — ½ — 1

N

TARR INLET

Russell
Island

1150'

2950'

3790'

3720'

Grand Pacific Glacier

CANADA
U.S.

Margerie Glacier

2190'

MAP 11

Chapter 12

TRIP 8 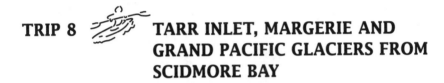 **TARR INLET, MARGERIE AND GRAND PACIFIC GLACIERS FROM SCIDMORE BAY**

Trip Details

Distance:	45 miles RT from Scidmore Bay drop-off
	43-mile tour from Rendu point campsite to Scidmore Bay drop-off
Time:	5-8 days
Rating:	Moderate to Difficult
Maps:	NOAA Chart 17318; USGS topos: Mt. Fairweather (D-2) & (D-3); Skagway (A-6)

Summary and Highlights

An intriguing part of this trip is floating in your kayak beneath the 200'-high face of Margerie Glacier, one of the most active ice flows in Glacier Bay. The sloughing of bus-sized bergs becomes commonplace, and you can get lucky—stay clear— when a house-sized one falls. Whale sightings around Russell Island are likely in the summer. Murres, marbled murrelets, and kittiwakes are often seen in Tarr Inlet. In addition, scaup, golden eye, and surf scoters sometimes raft together in large numbers in the bay east of Russell Island. Hazards include the ever-present cold water, and the sudden occurrence of glacial winds. Wind waves can be a hazard here, too, especially on the channel crossings.

Area Features, Background, and Tips

With Muir Glacier in rapid retreat and unapproachable by water during the early part of this century, Margerie and Grand Pacific Glaciers became the cruise ship destination in Glacier Bay. Ice had covered the inlet to Russell Island until 1892. By 1907 Grand Pacific had retreated to within 3 miles of its present location, face beside face with its former tributary, Margerie Glacier. Grand Pacific has been fickle: in 1920 it receded nearly 2 miles north into Canada, but by 1948 it had advanced to the U.S. border. The present face is nearly a mile south of the border. Grand Pacific Glacier ice is streaked with gravel and mud, probably as a result of its melding with soiled Ferris Glacier a mile north of the border. As a result, the dirty ice of Grand Pacific hardly receives a second glance.

If Grand Pacific is dingy, Margerie Glacier is largely sparkling white. Since Grand Pacific retreated north to reveal it, Margerie Glacier today is the crown jewel of tidewater glaciers. Other rivals are less active, like Lamplugh, or unapproachable because of ice, like Johns Hopkins. Margerie reliably presents—at least in the short term—an imposing, 200'-high face which calves frequently into deep water.

The west arm of Glacier Bay is windier than other parts of the fiord system. Broad waterways offer the winds an open sweep. Also, the Fairweather Range's eastern slopes spawn a southeasterly flow of air which in cooling pours down off the many icefields and glaciers. In the western arm of Glacier Bay and especially Tarr Inlet, you must be prepared to deal with this glacial wind, particularly during periods of clear weather. Floating ice is frequently

Face of Margerie Glacier from Tarr Inlet

encountered in Tarr Inlet, as far south as Russell Island. Bergs from Johns Hopkins Inlet and Lamplugh Glacier, both just 4 miles west of Russell Island, can be encountered anywhere in northwest Glacier Bay.

While there are numerous points and coves that offer protection for paddlers if the wind becomes too strong in Glacier Bay or Tarr Inlet, there are also shoreline sections which offer no protection for several miles. Paddling these exposed stretches of water should be done with care, preferably when it is calm, and sudden, strong winds are least likely to occur. Mornings are often preferable to afternoons in this regard. Generally, the shorelines of Glacier Bay from Composite Island north are steep. Exceptions are along the mainland shore east of Russell Island, and the large outwash fans on the west shore of Tarr Inlet 5 miles north of Russell. The west shore of Russell Island itself also slopes gently. It is possible to camp at the north end of Russell. Streams enter Tarr Inlet every mile or so, making drinking water easy to obtain. Nearer the head of the inlet, streams can be clouded with glacial silt. Since water may not be available at the spot you want to camp, you should bring some with you.

In this tourist-frequented section of Glacier Bay, paddlers will usually see two large cruise ships each day, the limit imposed by the Park Service. These ships normally cruise mid-channel in the waterways. When they are weaving through ice packs, near Margerie Glacier for instance, cruise ships can maneuver closer to shore. A few smaller ships—vessels to 200 feet in length that carry a limited number of passengers—will probably appear. Smaller still are some eco-tour ships, and the daily, park tour boat. Strict daily limits keep the traffic within reason. Your encounter with all these vessels is usually at long range. Still, under the right wind conditions, these vessels' wakes can be large.

Trip Description

Begin Trip 8 either as a continuation of Trip 7 to Rendu, Queen, and Tidal inlets, or take the park tour boat to the Scidmore Bay drop-off. If you begin at the Scidmore drop-off, you will need to cross Glacier Bay. From the drop-off point, head 2 miles north to that point on the north shore that is 1 mile west of the peninsula tip dividing the main bay and Rendu Inlet (Map 9). If such a crossing seems daunting to you, you could paddle Trip 9 in reverse from the Scidmore drop-off, thereby remaining on the west side of Glacier Bay. At the north end of Trip 9 you could paddle up Tarr Inlet, and then return by the same route to the Scidmore pickup.

Consistent with a counterclockwise circumnavigation of Glacier Bay, Trip 8 starts at the cove 1 mile west of the peninsula tip dividing Rendu Inlet from the main bay. This cove provides good camping on a level bench near a stream. Leave the cove and paddle 4 miles northwest along a shoreline which offers little shelter and few landing possibilities, to a sizable stream which flows into the bay (Map 10). Directly opposite, 0.7 mile offshore, is a cluster of tiny islands. These are part of a submerged ridge, and submerged rocks and islets offshore dot a line for 4 miles to the midpoint of Russell Island. Near the stream the shoreline becomes gentler, and there are many gravel and shingle beaches. There are also a number of brown bears that include this stretch of beach in their foraging area.

Continue 2 miles beyond the stream, passing two small creeks along the way, to the entrance of another larger stream. This flow drains an unseen lake tucked in a cirque some 2500 feet above. Now the channel between Russell Island and the mainland begins to narrow. At the same time, the mainland beach becomes flatter, with gravel and shingle stretches for hauling out. Alder is thick ashore, in a dense strip just back from the beach. This is a good area for sea ducks; depending upon the season you may see hundreds of scaup, golden eye, or surf scoters here. The channel northeast of Russell Island is classified as whale waters, but it does not restrict kayakers.

Paddle 3 miles up the inlet from the last stream, to the narrowest part of the channel between Russell Island's east point and the gravel outwash fans on your right. These tidal flats, created by streams draining the west slopes of Mt. Abdallah, reduce the channel's width to a few hundred yards. No one knows how long it will be before alluvium and mud block this passage entirely, turning Russell Island into a peninsula.

From the east point, paddle along the northeast shore of Russell Island for 1 mile, then leave the north tip behind and cut over to the northeast mainland shore. Several seasonal streams enter along the north side of an outwash which has created a shallow cove 1 mile north of Russell (11 miles from the Rendu Pt. cove). Here a rounded point provides some protection should down-channel breezes kick up.

From just off the rounded point, if you look north up Tarr Inlet you'll get the first glimpse of Margerie and Grand Pacific glaciers (Map 11). The glacier faces—nearly 8 miles distant—appear much closer than they actually are. You may encounter your first icebergs at close range here. Ebb-tide currents move bergs south down the inlet; when the tide turns and the current reverses, the flood pushes them back. Salt water is tough on bergs, melting them quickly.

From the shallow cove, paddle 2 miles north of the rounded point to the inflow of a sizable stream, which originates in glacier remnants to the east at 4000 feet in elevation. The shore describes a gently concave arc here, ending 2 miles northwest of the stream at a broad outwash formed by another, glacial-flour-filled stream. There is a shallow cove 1 mile north of this outwash, where camping is possible above a shingle beach.

When you are 1 mile farther north, the large, rocky point dominating Tarr Inlet's west shore is directly across from you. Ice can be thick from this point on. Generally there are more open leads along the east shore, as Margerie Glacier calves on the west shore. The east shore ends in tidal flats 5 miles beyond the shallow cove. On the east shore near the flats, a small, rocky point marks one of several possible campsites (21 miles from the Rendu pt.cove). Before you camp here, consider that your departure should coincide with open water lanes, especially if calving has been very active. Since Margerie is a noisy glacier, your stay here will be punctuated with many pops and groans, and the periodic, thunder-like reports of ice falling into the water.

Grand Pacific Glacier will mutter too, with occasional, thunderous calving. Most of the bergs you see, however, will be from ever-active Margerie. Even on breezy days, you can drift and observe Margerie Glacier. Watch one or two huge bergs topple into the water, and you won't want to get closer than the one-quarter mile recommended for safety. Sheer cliffs at Margerie Glacier's south end are used as a rookery by a large colony of black-legged kittiwakes. With yellow bills, black legs, and wing tips that look as if they had been dipped in ink, these otherwise white gulls congregate here each season to raise their young. The cruise ships, which you will surely encounter in Tarr Inlet, can be 700 to 800 feet in length. Pilots are busy watching the bergs and the ship's position. A kayak may, or may not, be seen. Don't even think about closely approaching cruise ships. At any time maneuvering can be necessary, which could create strong currents and swirling bergs. Respect the right of ships to be there, and their crews will respect you.

You will probably leave the area around Margerie Glacier along the east shore, because of the ice. If you are retracing the route paddled on the way north, stay along the east shore. From Margerie Glacier it is 23 miles to the Scidmore Bay pickup. Along the west shore 2 miles south of Margerie Glacier, a bay is formed by the prominent rocky point. Ice tends to congregate around this bay, and the area is unprotected from glacial winds. Camping here is possible if you can tolerate these two disadvantages to what would otherwise be a spectacular campsite. If the ice is thick, paddle south before trying to work your way across to the west shore of the inlet. At the south end of the blunt, rocky point—1 mile from its north end—a small, hooked point forms a protected cove where you can camp. If ice prevents you from reaching this point, paddle south 2.5 miles to another hooked point on the west shore just south of an inflow stream. Camping and shelter can be found in the cove south of this point. (26.5 miles from the Rendu pt. cove).

South of this cove the shoreline is steep, with cliffs and talus jumbles that make landing very difficult. Paddle 2.5 miles south to another small cove cut into the broad peninsula at its easternmost extent (Map 12). Landing and camping are possible here. If you are continuing into Johns Hopkins Inlet, keep to the west shore of Tarr Inlet until you round the peninsula. The shore is steep and rocky—not at all hospitable—with only a few places to land if absolutely necessary. Continue 1.5 miles south to the southern point of the peninsula. There are possible campsites within the first 0.2 mile west of the point (31 miles from the Rendu Pt. cove). From this camp you are poised to begin Trip 9. Or, if you have chosen to return to the North Scidmore Bay pickup along this route, the pickup point is approximately 12 miles southeast, excluding explorations into Johns Hopkins and Reid inlets.

⊷ ⊨◊⊨ ⊶

Has the wind stopped? Are there any bears near the food canisters? Arising at 2:00 A.M. puts thoughts like these in our heads. We are camped in a snug cove 3 miles west of Composite Island, where yesterday's impossible wind and waves ended our progress. Outside the tent, the usual half-light made brighter by a full moon lets us see out into the main bay. There are no whitecaps visible, and no sounds of wind waves crashing onto shore. The wind has abated; this will be our day in Tarr Inlet.

We cut a half hour off the time it usually takes to make breakfast, break camp, and load the boat. By 3:00 A.M. we have rounded the point, and are on our way toward Russell Island. In sliding down toward the Fairweathers, the full moon's

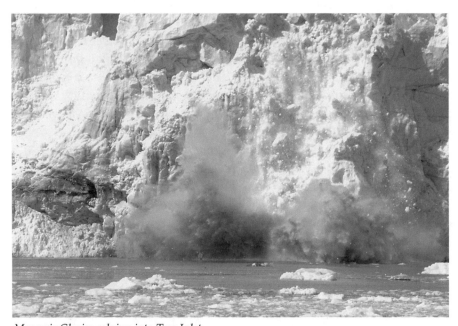

Margerie Glacier calving into Tarr Inlet

icy disk paints a shimmering strip on the otherwise black water. Poor light prevents us from seeing into the water, so we stay away from shore to avoid rocks.

The whoosh of a surfacing humpback momentarily startles us, and when we look over our shoulders, two more whales surface behind us. Out come our cameras. When the whales breathe again, they are lit in the moonbeam, and our cameras click. These are the three we encountered near Composite Island two days ago; now travelling fast northwest toward Tarr Inlet. We put our cameras back into water-proof storage, pick up our paddles, and get underway. Suddenly we are in the mid-dle of a huge, black boil: water welling up beneath us, all around our 20' boat. But there is no contact; the whale has merely come to check us out. Invisible in the black water, the creature sounded as we paddled above it, the rolling boil nearly scaring us out of the kayak. We sit for a few minutes—hearts thumping—before we can resume paddling.

It is fully light by 4:00 A.M. when we reach Russell Island, the much larger cousin to small islets and submerged rocks we've been passing. The ebb tide slows our progress through the island's narrow, northeast channel before releasing us to the lazier currents at Tarr Inlet's mouth. The face of Margerie Glacier is suddenly visible, a shimmering wall of white ice which seems only 2 or 3 miles away, but which our chart says is at the head of Tarr Inlet, nearly 9 miles distant. As we pad-dle, the rays of the sun extend to the white ice, setting reflective fire to the ice cliffs.

The first bergs, larger than those in Muir Inlet, float by on their daily sashay up and down the inlet. And now we hear what we at first take to be thunder. But there is not a cloud in the sky; nothing except mountains to reflect in the glassy surface dotted now with numerous bergs. Then we realize that the thunder is the glacier's voicing of internal stress: the explosive reports of bergs calved into the inlet. The glacier face reflects the sound, projecting it out over the inlet like an amplifier.

By 9:00 A.M. we are drifting silently, 500 yards from the face of Margerie Glacier. Careful maneuvering between bergs has enabled us to reach this spot. Above us, the nearly 200'-high face of Margerie sparkles in the sun. Bus-sized blocks tumble down without warning, accompanied by smaller chunks and a dump-truck load of slush. The booming splash reverberates, and a minute or so later our boat, a quarter mile from the face, rocks in a gentle rings-on-a-pond wave. Then complete calm returns to the glassy surface. While Grand Pacific Glacier also mutters, booms and calves, it is less impressive, the face dirtied with silt and grav-el. At low tide, ice blocks fall into mud, waiting to be lifted on the flood. But Margerie Glacier steals the show.

Around 10:00 A.M. the cruise ship which we've been watching for an hour finally threads its way through the bergs and takes a front-and-center station along Margerie Glacier. We photograph this floating city, and contemplate its passengers' perspective compared to ours. The ship moves slowly, coming between us and the glacier. We withdraw—backing, turning—careful of the bergs around us. On the ship, all passengers are facing the glacial spectacle. Then we see them, four people standing amidship on an upper deck, facing our way. Through our binoculars, we see they are looking at us through theirs. We wave, and on the ship four arms go up in response. Then our kayak is weaving south among the bergs.

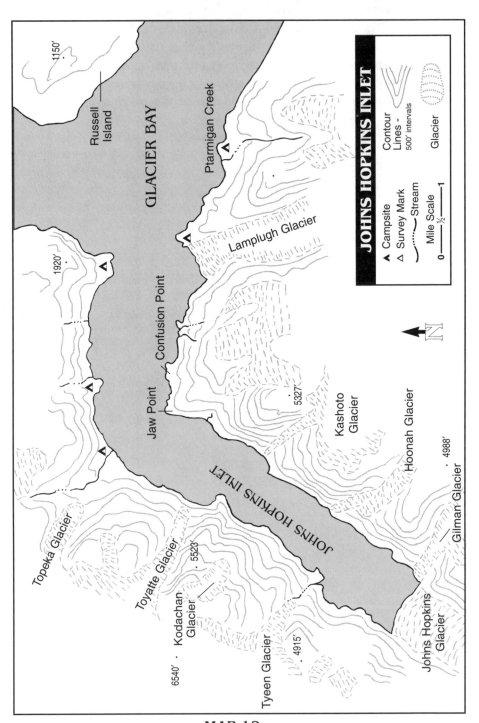

JOHNS HOPKINS INLET

▲ Campsite
△ Survey Mark
Contour
Lines -
500' intervals
——— Stream
Glacier

Mile Scale
0   ½   1

GLACIER BAY

Russell
Island

1150'

1920'

Ptarmigan Creek

Lamplugh Glacier

Confusion Point

Jaw Point

5327'

Kashoto
Glacier

Hoonah Glacier

4988'

Gilman Glacier

JOHNS HOPKINS INLET

Topeka Glacier

Toyatte Glacier

Kodachan
Glacier

6540'

5523'

Tyeen Glacier

4915'

Johns Hopkins
Glacier

N

MAP 12

Chapter 13

TRIP 9 **JOHNS HOPKINS AND REID INLETS FROM SCIDMORE BAY**

Trip Details

Distance:	24 miles RT from Scidmore Bay drop-off
	20 miles from Tarr-Johns Hopkins peninsula campsite to Scidmore Bay pickup
Time:	3-5 days
Rating:	Moderate
Maps:	NOAA Chart 17318; USGS Topos: Mt. Fairweather (D-3) & (D-4)

Summary and Highlights

Johns Hopkins Inlet, and its glaciers, are without a doubt the most stunning area in Glacier Bay. The steep canyon walls, viewed from kayak level, seem to rise forever upward. While some smaller glaciers reach the inlet, a few do not, holding to precarious slopes and sending silt-stream feelers down to tidewater. The inlet is usually choked with ice. Southwest of Jaw Point, Johns Hopkins Inlet is closed to cruise ships from May 1 to August 31, and to all other vessels including kayaks from May 1 to June 30 due to seals pupping on the ice. The Ibach Cabin at Reid Inlet will remind you of the colorful couple that lived there. The cabin is one of few relics left within the park from earlier mining operations. Brown bears are plentiful in the area covered by this trip. Hazards include the extremely cold water, and the ice pack which can make navigation impossible when it is thick. Glacial winds can burst suddenly out into the inlets, creating waves and concentrating ice.

Area Features, Background, and Tips

Johns Hopkins Inlet is probably more memorable to kayakers than any portion of Glacier Bay's west arm. If the ever-present ice is not impressive enough, the visual impact of a mile-wide fiord flanked by steep canyon walls rising to over 7000 feet commands attention. It is an inlet of gray rock, snow, ice fields, and at least five glaciers, three of which reach tidewater. Johns Hopkins Glacier, at the inlet head, is a product of four or five huge, octopus-like, glacial arms joining in a single flow. It is a very active glacier, which has been advancing since 1929. This advance has progressed to the point that, in 1997, Johns Hopkins and Gilman glaciers are nearly joined. Your topo map will show them a mile apart. Johns Hopkins has been much studied, and during its current, 50-year advance, has yielded a lot of information to glaciologists.

Advancing tidewater glaciers push ahead of them a gravelly underwater shoal, or plug, formed as the glacier simultaneously bulldozes forward, and deposits rock and silt from its melting face. The plug protects the large, underwater portion of the glacier from salt-water exposure, thereby slowing the melting process and enabling the glacier to advance. Between the top of the plug and the surface of tidewater, melting takes place at a rate more rapid than if the ice were exposed to air. The result is undercutting, leaving the outer

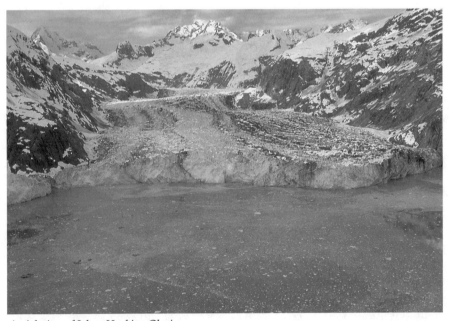

Aerial view of Johns Hopkins Glacier

face unsupported below. Lack of support for that part of the face above the waterline is what causes calving. In Johns Hopkins Inlet, the water depth is around 1200 feet until you approach the glacier face. Abrupt shoaling there betrays the presence of the submarine plug.

One current theory explaining why glaciers advance or recede hinges on the altitude of the ice mass which feeds them. In the case of Johns Hopkins, the huge, ice-field sources lie at an average elevation above 6000 feet. These high, ice fields are on the east slope of the coastal ridge, where moisture is squeezed from Pacific storms by Fairweather Range peaks up to 15,000 feet in elevation. A large amount of snow falls here, increasing the thickness of the ice fields which feed the glaciers. Ice fields feeding Muir and other, east-arm glaciers lie at a much lower elevation, around 3000 feet. Since the precipitation is less at these locations, there is less snow to replenish the ice fields. Most, if not all, of the east-arm glaciers are presently receding. In all likelihood they will continue their retreat until some prolonged period of climatic change increases the snowfall accumulation in their ice-field sources.

Johns Hopkins Inlet has become the choice location for hundreds of birthing harbor seals in Glacier Bay. Biologists think that this is a learned response to the ideal conditions offered by the sheltering ice. Killer whales, or orcas, rarely enter the upper portions of Glacier Bay inlets, possibly because the silty water may disable their natural sonar capabilities. Freedom from this major predator, with little or no disturbance from humans, may be the reason seals come to the ice floes in Johns Hopkins to pup.

To protect seals from disturbance during the critical time from birth until the pups are a few weeks old, the Park Service imposes a closure on boating within the inlet beyond Jaw Point from May 1 to June 30 for all boats, and extends the closure for cruise ships until August 31. Between July 1 and August 31, all vessels including kayaks must remain one-quarter mile from any seals hauled out on the ice. The large amount of ice present in Johns Hopkins Inlet often renders the boating regulations moot. Yet, conditions vary with the season and the particular year, and at certain times it is possible to paddle most of the way through the ice pack to the proximity of the glacier face.

On the south shore 3 miles east of Jaw Point, Lamplugh Glacier calves into tidewater. This glacier is receding at a slow rate. A current shoreline indentation of 0.5 mile hints at the future unveiling of an inlet. A 500' water depth just a few hundred meters from the face suggests that an inlet lies, ready-carved, beneath the glacier.

Reid Inlet, one of the more colorful spots in Glacier Bay's brief history, lies 4 miles east. Sometime prior to 1940, Joe Ibach, a prospector, discovered gold in the ridges between Reid Inlet and Ptarmigan Creek. In 1940, he and his wife, Muz, built a small cabin on a spit at the west entrance to Reid Inlet, seasonally occupying this spot until 1959. Several large spruce trees now growing beside the cabin owe their existence to being transplanted by the Ibachs, giving the spruce an ecological headstart. But there was little gold and much work; one can speculate that the benefits of summers spent at Reid Inlet were largely aesthetic rather than monetary. Muz planted a garden, using soil that had to be hauled in. Standing at the spot today, you can experience some of the sights they saw. But not all. When Harry Reid, an early glaciologist, mapped Glacier Bay, Reid Inlet was completely entombed in ice. In 1940, Reid Glacier had retreated only as far as the south toe of the small point where the Ibachs built their cabin. Its face must have been an imposing presence, undoubtedly overshadowing all other landscape features.

In 1997, Reid Inlet is 2.5 miles long, with Reid Glacier sometimes advancing, sometimes receding at the head. The inlet is quite shallow between the entrance points, but deepens to 180 feet near the center. Shoaling again occurs near the glacier's face. If receding continues, Reid Glacier will soon become grounded. Both Reid and Lamplugh glaciers are tongues of the huge Brady Icefield, occupying half of the area of the entire peninsula south of the Fairweather Range. Certainly there is adequate precipitation at that location to support the active glaciers which flow from the Brady. Who knows what subtle changes over time may cause these tidewater glaciers to begin a steady advance?

Trip Description

This adventure is an ideal extension of the Tarr Inlet paddle (Trip 8) described in Chapter 12. As such, Trip 9 will be described starting just west of the southern tip of the peninsula dividing Tarr and Johns Hopkins inlets. If you are paddling Trip 9 starting at the Scidmore Bay drop-off, merely follow the directions in reverse.

From the campsite just west of the southern tip of the peninsula dividing Tarr and Johns Hopkins inlets, paddle 1.5 miles west to a tiny cove formed by an equally small point (Map 12). Some shelter may be found here. From the small point, paddle 1 mile west to a larger point. Landing and camping is possible here. This second point shunts ice away from the north shore, often creating an open channel to paddle. Circumnavigate this point for a breathtaking view of Johns Hopkins Glacier and the upper inlet, a sight you will never forget.

Beyond this point, the inlet turns gradually to the southwest. If the ice will let you, paddle 1.5 miles west to the beginning of the large, gravel outwash fan from Topeka Glacier (4 miles from the Tarr-Johns Hopkins peninsula campsite). Landing and camping are possible here, but like most of Johns Hopkins Inlet, snow may blanket much of the shore until late summer. At Topeka Glacier, you are less than 1.5 miles from the boating closure line which runs due west from Jaw Point. Up inlet from this area there are few campsites, even if you are visiting in late season after the waters open to boating.

From the Topeka Glacier fan, paddle 1.2 miles southeast to Jaw Point. This crossing can involve a difficult time with pack ice. If crossing here is not feasible, retrace your route along the north shore of the inlet to the last sheltering point; then cross the inlet to Confusion Point, which is 1 mile east of Jaw Point. Ice density and wind conditions are the factors that determine the difficulty of channel crossings here. If you are able to cross to Jaw Point, you will be reeling under the impact of unforgettable views. From Jaw Point, turn east and paddle 3 miles to Lamplugh Glacier, passing a meltwater stream at the midpoint which drains a glacier hanging some 2500 feet above you. While there are a few, cramped campsites near small haulouts along this reach, better camping awaits you at Lamplugh Glacier.

At Lamplugh Glacier's east point, you can land near the tip, and camp on top of the rocky knolls and ledges there (9 miles from the Tarr-Johns Hopkins peninsula campsite). Your sleep will be punctuated by the grumblings and calving booms which echo from Lamplugh's face. Ice can collect in the Lamplugh cove, and also in the cove just west of Ptarmigan Creek. Pay attention to the winds and tides while in this area to prevent being surrounded unexpectedly by ice. The entrance to Ptarmigan Creek is 2 miles east of Lamplugh's east point (Map 10). There are good gravel beaches by the creek. This is a popular camping area, and one of the few places where you can see relics of mining activity in the park. An old mining road, now little more than an overgrown trail, was constructed up Ptarmigan Creek.

From Ptarmigan Creek, paddle 2.5 miles east along the curve of the shoreline to the west point marking the mouth of Reid Inlet. The point is well inside the inlet and somewhat protected from down-bay winds. The Ibach Cabin, with its attendant spruce trees, hard to miss. This, too, is a popular spot to camp, because of the glacial views. Reid Glacier is just 2 miles south. Just 0.7 mile east, across the inlet, you can find good camping on Ibach Point and the adjoining beach. Hiking is easier around Reid Inlet than at many locations within the bay. The alder is either low and scattered, or can easily be avoided; and the terrain offers several plausible routes to elevated points for views of the bay.

From the Ibach Cabin point, paddle 2 miles south to Reid Glacier. While not nearly as active as Johns Hopkins or Lamplugh glaciers, Reid still moans, groans, and occasionally calves bergs into the inlet. Campsites can be found at the head of the inlet, on lateral moraine gravel at either side of the glacier face. Retrace the 2-mile paddle from Reid Glacier to Ibach Point. Continue 1 mile east of Ibach Point to a cove defined by a small point, where a sizable stream enters. The half-mile-long beach here offers good camping, with an extra

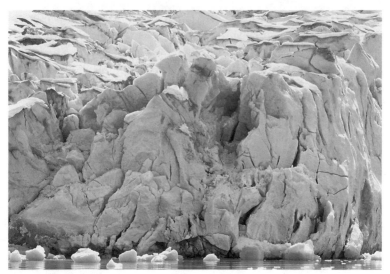

Snout of Reid Glacier

bonus: views of Grand Pacific Glacier northeast in Tarr Inlet, as well as the Fairweather Range to the west.

Paddle 3 miles southeast of the long beach, parallel to the rocky coast with few haul-outs, to another wide, gravel beach. A stream, which is the outlet for a lake 1 mile south in the draw, enters here (21 miles from the Tarr-Johns Hopkins peninsula campsite). The Scidmore Bay pickup is located near this stream during the early season when salmon aren't spawning here. Later in the summer, the pickup point is moved approximately 3 miles southeast, near the north, tidal channel entrance to Scidmore Bay. Verify the pickup point location at the park headquarters before you set out.

━━ ━◆━ ━━

There is something different about Johns Hopkins Inlet, a feeling of foreboding, that we can't identify. The physical splendor around us belies it and entices us; we're eager to experience this stunning, ice-choked fiord with gray-and-white, confining walls towering above us. Yet, bergs and slush ice in the water demand care, since the route we paddle can close behind us. We're being drawn by the spectacle of rock walls split by icy, glacial tongues, but unlike the other experiences we've had in Glacier Bay, we have a feeling that unknown conditions in this inlet can turn on us.

Breaking indiscriminately through overcast skies, a weak sun distinguishes some near-vertical slopes. In May the ice fields and glaciers are still blanketed with snow down to the tideline. The chilled air is still, and there's silence except for the ice groans and the distant booming of calving bergs. Johns Hopkins draws us, as if to the brink of a waterfall's edge. We can't resist paddling as far as the ice will allow—our adrenaline coursing.

Then we can paddle no farther. To open leads requires pushing against bergs, something we avoid. The route there can close behind us without warning. Ahead the inlet is closed to boating because of seal pupping. We back and jockey the kayak around, threading our retreat through narrow passages, and finally, into more open water. A physical barrier—the ice—stopped us short of the administrative one.

We drift for a while, sorting out our ambivalent feelings. We have never seen so much ice, nor have we seen an inlet cradled in so deep and narrow a canyon. We are reduced to a feeling of insignificance that demands awe and respect. This, we decide, is the attraction. And yet that same raw, rugged beauty and omnipotence that attracts, projects a warning to us, as humans, to pass through warily and with reverence or not at all.

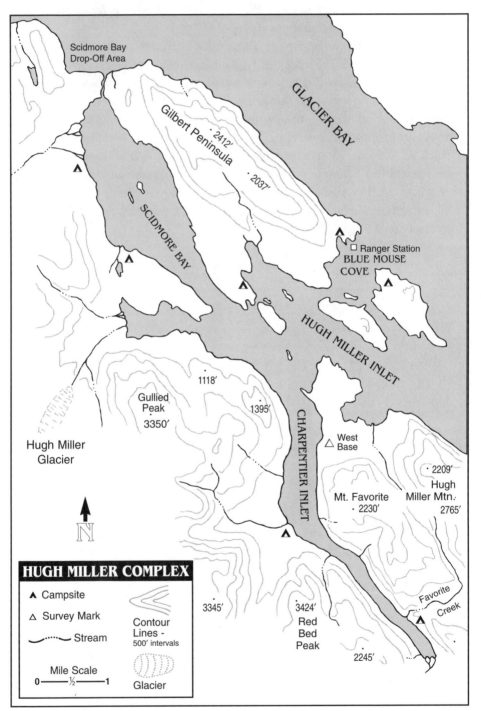

Scidmore Bay
Drop-Off Area

GLACIER BAY

Gilbert Peninsula
· 2412'
· 2037'

SCIDMORE BAY

□ Ranger Station
BLUE MOUSE
COVE

HUGH MILLER INLET

· 1118'

Gullied
Peak
·
3350'

· 1395'

CHARPENTIER INLET

Hugh Miller
Glacier

△ West
Base

· 2209'
Hugh
Miller Mtn.
2765'

Mt. Favorite
· 2230'

N

· 3345'

· 3424'
Red
Bed
Peak

Favorite
Creek

· 2245'

HUGH MILLER COMPLEX

▲ Campsite

△ Survey Mark

⌁ Stream

Contour
Lines -
500' intervals

Mile Scale
0 — ½ — 1

Glacier

MAP 13

Chapter 14

TRIP 10   SCIDMORE BAY TO BLUE MOUSE COVE VIA CHARPENTIER AND HUGH MILLER INLETS

Trip Details

Distance:	50 miles RT from Scidmore Bay drop-off
	35 miles from Scidmore Bay drop-off ending at Blue Mouse Cove
Time:	5-7 days
Rating:	Easy to Moderate
Maps:	NOAA chart 17318; USGS topos: Mt. Fairweather (C-2) & (D-2)

Summary and Highlights

This trip visits a bay and inlet complex that lies west of the west arm of Glacier Bay. These protected waters offer many miles of pleasant paddling in a secluded estuary. Camping opportunities abound. The complex is off-limits to motorized boats from May 15 to September 15, with the exception of Blue Mouse Cove. A park ranger is present at a floating station in Blue Mouse Cove during the peak season. This protected estuary complex rivals Adams Inlet as a favorite destination for kayakers. Your hazards here are cold water, current in the narrow channels, and wind waves arising when glacial winds sweep down the inlet.

Area Features, Background, and Tips

Blue Mouse Cove lies just north of Hugh Miller Inlet, separated from it by two islands. The cove is a favorite anchorage for private vessels because it

123

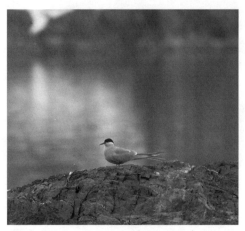

Arctic terns congregate in the protected estuary west of Scidmore Bay

allows access to intimate places, being shallow enough for anchorage, yet deep enough to avoid stranding. There are few such anchorages in Glacier Bay. To accommodate private vessels and the floating ranger station there, Blue Mouse Cove is outside the non-motorized area.

The large volume of tidewater in Charpentier Inlet and Scidmore Bay ebbs and flows through constricted passages between Charpentier and Hugh Miller inlets. A long, hooked-shaped peninsula with several trailing islets effectively narrows this channel so much that current velocities can exceed the speed at which you are able to paddle. At these times small swirls and rips are present. Skirt around these high velocity formations. You will have no trouble seeing them as you approach. Similar currents exists in a passage leading to the idyllic, unnamed estuary which lies west of the entrance to Scidmore Bay. A very narrow channel leads northwest into the estuary. Flows through this channel during mid-flood and ebb tides can create small whirlpools and rips, so make your entrance and exit "going with the flow," or near the time of slack water.

This small, westside estuary is a special place. It is completely protected from the prevailing winds of Glacier Bay. At its western head is the 0.7-mile-wide outwash from Hugh Miller Glacier, whose stream braids various channels, sometimes meandering across the entire width of the gravel fan. The calm waters may be the reason that many hundreds of waterfowl congregate here, especially in midsummer. The birds seek out sheltered areas in which to pass time during their flightless molting season.

Scidmore Bay was named for Eliza Scidmore, a writer who was inspired by John Muir's accounts to visit Glacier Bay in the 1880s. Her description of calving glaciers, and the raw beauty of Glacier Bay at that time, is still vivid today. In 1880, only Blue Mouse Cove and the southern portion of Hugh Miller Inlet had emerged from the ice. Some 12 years later, the ice had receded to the mouths of Scidmore Bay and Charpentier Inlet. The latter inlet was being unzipped from each end, with the glacier retreating entirely from the midriff section around 1920. During the two decades after 1900, Hugh Miller Glacier alternately receded and advanced. By 1907 it had advanced and again covered a small portion of its inlet. But overall it was a period of retreat, and 15 years later the bays and inlets of the Hugh Miller complex were free of ice.

Alignment of these estuaries clearly demonstrates that the major glacial sculpturing was accomplished by Grand Pacific Glacier, now grounded to the northwest at the head of Tarr Inlet. Including tributary Melbourne Glacier, Grand Pacific maintains its northwest-southeast alignment for some 30 miles into Canada. Hugh Miller and Scidmore glaciers had little overall effect other than minor, westside gouging. Gilbert Peninsula and its attendant islands reveal striations and gouging left from their most recent glacial reshaping.

Charpentier Inlet is unique in being the narrowest waterway of appreciable size within Glacier Bay. The precipitous slopes of Red Bed Peak border the southwest shore, while the cliffs and ledges of Mt. Favorite wall in the other side of this narrow fiord. A sizable waterfall display on the west shore is attractive for paddlers.

Trip Description

If you are paddling this trip as a continuation of a completed trip through Johns Hopkins and Reid inlets to the north, you are already at the Scidmore Bay drop-off point. Begin Trip 10 at this drop-off point, which in early season is near the mouth of a stream 4 miles east of Ibach Point (Map 10). Check the drop-off location at park headquarters because it may change during the season. Paddle 2 miles east to the S-shaped tidal channel leading south into Scidmore Bay (Map 13). Since this is only a high-tide passage, plan your arrival or be prepared to wait. The alternative, 6-mile paddle around the rugged Gilbert Peninsula to the mouth of Blue Mouse Cove provides little protection from the elements and few haul-outs.

Paddle 0.3 mile through the narrow tidal channel into Scidmore Bay. Head 1 mile southeast to the extensive gravel fan formed by meltwater from Scidmore Glacier. Camping is good on either side of the outwash fan, but the south side may be better; it has excellent views north to the mouths of Rendu and Queen inlets. There is some alder here, but stretches of gravel provide open areas for your tent. Continue 2 miles south from the outwash, following the gravel beach forming the west shore of the bay. Just beyond a shallow cove at the end of a long beach, a small stream enters the bay. There are camping possibilities near this stream, which drains a series of small lakes to the south. From the stream, head 2 miles southeast to the entrance of the bay. This paddle is along a steep, rocky shoreline with few places to land and no good places to camp.

Go around the western peninsula at the entrance to Scidmore Bay; then head 0.5 mile west toward the estuary which lies a short distance inland. At lower water levels, the estuary passage is obscured by a mile-wide, gravelly tidal flat. The narrow channel is just north of the center of this tidal flat. Turn northwest into the channel, and paddle 0.6 mile through this slit. If the tide is rising, you will be carried along. If the ebb tide is in mid-flow, you will probably have to wait, as few kayakers can paddle against this current.

Once inside the estuary, you will find that both shores are comprised of tidal flats. There is camping near the west end, 1 mile from the entrance channel, on both sides of the gravel outwash from Hugh Miller Glacier. The north shore of the estuary is low lying, with flats covered with dryas. To the south, though, the impressive slopes of Gullied Peak rise up sharply behind gravel beaches. One drawback to camping in this calm, bird sanctuary is that the water recedes a long way from your camp at low tide. It is also difficult to camp here at all without disturbing the birds, especially during their molt.

Retracing your route out of the estuary is best done on an ebb or slack tide because of channel current. Once out of the channel, paddle 2 miles southeast to the mouth of Charpentier Inlet, passing a shallow bay with submerged rocks along the shoreline. Charpentier Inlet is barely defined by a rounded point on the west. Paddle 2 miles south of the point along a steep, shoreline—now heavily forested—to the first of several streams entering on the right. When you are 1.5 miles south of the stream, you pass a 0.7-mile-wide cove which is filled by mud flats. These flats result from the combined outwash from Charpentier and Maynard glaciers. Fair campsites can be found on the gravel fan.

Continue 1 mile south of the outwash to where a small, rounded point narrows Charpentier Inlet to barely one-quarter mile wide. You will hear a waterfall just beyond this point before you see it. The flow forms impressive cascades as it falls the last 700-800' to the water. From the waterfall, paddle 3 miles south along the narrow, forested inlet to its head (21 miles from the Scidmore Bay drop-off). A stream draining 3500' Mt. Bulky to the west enters here. Strangely, a closely parallel stream from the same watershed turns and flows south into Geikie Inlet. Mudflats and the low shoreline at Charpentier Inlet head make for poor camping.

For a better campsite, paddle 1 mile north along the east shore to Favorite Creek. The forest ends north of here, giving way on the east shore to the bare, steep slopes of Mt. Favorite. With seemingly vertical walls on either side of the narrow fiord, you feel closed in along this section. From Favorite Creek, paddle 4 miles north along the base of the near-vertical shoreline, to a rounded point across from the Charpentier Glacier outwash. Paddle 2 miles north along this arrow-straight shore, to several shallow coves near the topo survey mark WEST BASE. From these coves go 1 mile north to a thin peninsula marking the start of a shallow area of mudflats, islets, and submerged rocks. Since a great thing about paddle boats is their ability to maneuver in shallow water, you can circumnavigate the narrow spit, and go 0.5 mile northeast.

Now, you are just east of the northernmost point of the Mt. Favorite peninsula, between Charpentier and Hugh Miller inlets. Projecting from this point is a large, hook-shaped bar, submerged at high water, that trails off to the east after 0.3 mile. Submerged rocks and an islet lie 100 yards farther east. At extreme low water, these features can blend together in one, big tidal flat: a significant extension of the peninsula. Northeast of this shoal is an area of very strong currents, generating small whirls and rips. Paddle through here at, or near, slack water. Or at least stay out of areas of the fastest currents.

Once clear of the hooked bar, cross 0.7-mile-wide Hugh Miller Inlet to the island forming the south boundary of Blue Mouse Cove. Paddle 1 mile northwest along the shore of this unnamed island to the northwest end. Then head east through the passage at the south tip of Gilbert Peninsula, into Blue Mouse Cove. It is 1.5 miles northeast to possible campsites near the floating ranger station. This station is moored in a cove just west of the point at the north entrance to Blue Mouse Cove. From the northern coves of Blue Mouse, paddle 1.5 miles southeast to the prominent cove on the west side of the 545'-high island (35 miles from the Scidmore Bay drop-off). Good campsites are found here. If you are taking Trip 11, this cove is a good takeoff point.

To reach the Scidmore Bay pickup, return to the north shore of Blue Mouse Cove, and paddle 1.5 miles southwest to the passage with the south boundary island. Bear west through the channel into the head of Hugh Miller Inlet.

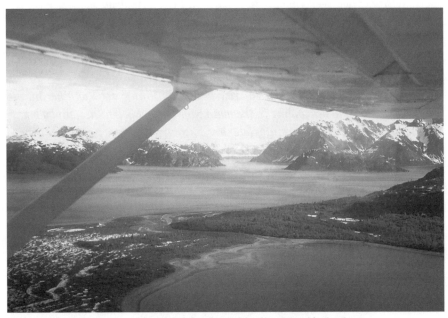

Over Scidmore Bay, an aerial view of the channel leading into Glacier Bay

Since this passage may be dry at low tide, either time your arrival for high water, or paddle around the island to enter the central portion of the inlet. Once through the island channel, upper Hugh Miller Inlet lies before you to explore. The inlet head isn't subjected to the strong tidal currents found between the central inlet and the entrance to Charpentier. Paddle 1.5 miles northwest to the head of the inlet, then go 0.5 mile south to a small, westshore cove with several islets. You can find campsites in this area if you spend a little time looking.

After a 0.5-mile paddle south of the cove, a channel leads west into Scidmore Bay between the peninsula and a small, 348'-high island. Go through this passage, and then paddle 2 miles north to two projecting points forming mini-coves along the east shore of Skidmore Bay. Then, paddle 4 miles north to the head of Scidmore Bay. Paddle out into Glacier Bay through the tidal passage, and go 2 miles northwest to the pickup point (50 miles round trip).

Glacial winds, and waves, made it easy to take the tidal channel shortcut. We reached smooth water by paddling just a few hundred yards through the shallow, rapidly-draining trough leading from Glacier Bay into the north end of Scidmore Bay. We drifted, allowing the wind and current to carry us slowly south, toward twin islands in the middle of the bay. Relief flooded over us. The paddle south to the tidal channel had been choppy, filling us with concern about making our passage before the tide ebbed, and transformed the channel into a mud flat. The sun moved toward the Fairweather Range behind us, gilding the snowy ridges with a shimmering fire; once extinguished, shadows crept out on the still water. Waterfowl flew by, heading south over a bay we had yet to explore.

Another beautiful day with skies a crisp blue. Continuing good weather means that glacial winds will be blowing in the main bay. We paddle south, round a point, and enter a narrow channel. Minutes later a strong current shoots us out into a magnificent, little estuarine bay. Hundreds of ducks, a few geese, countless gulls, and many Arctic terns are present here. Near the gravel outwash, a northern harrier engages in its seemingly erratic hunting patrol. We paddle slowly, keeping our distance from the avian residents. Our exit is made easy by a just-beginning ebb flow.

We are paddling down Charpentier Inlet, entering a section where the inlet narrows to a confining one-quarter mile wide. The sound of falling water intrigues us, but we can't see the source. Beyond a small point, a waterfall cascades from rock shelves and tumbles, taking major drops, down sections of the slender fiord's west wall. The roar is mostly absorbed by the dense forest, but the visual impact is deafening. We drift and take it in before paddling away.

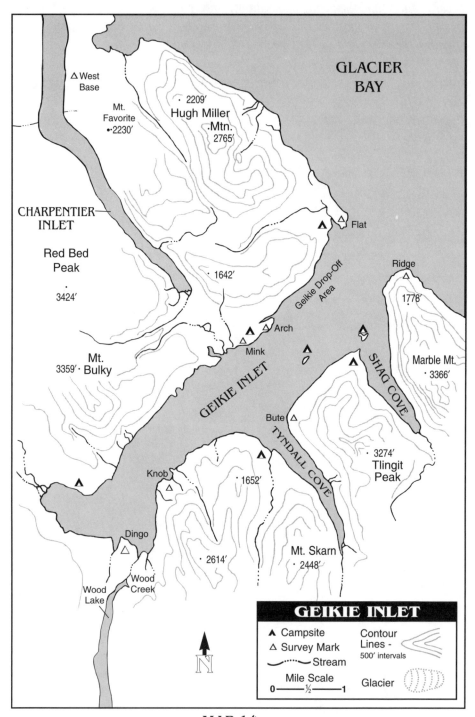

MAP 14

Chapter 15

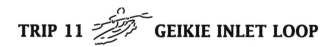

TRIP 11   GEIKIE INLET LOOP

Trip Details

Distance:	25 miles RT from Geikie Inlet drop-off
	10.5 miles from Blue Mouse Cove to Geikie Inlet pickup
Time:	3-5 days
Rating:	Easy
Maps:	NOAA chart 17318; USGS Topos: Mt. Fairweather (C-1) & (C-2)

Summary and Highlights

The vegetation at Geikie Inlet is older than that at other inlets to the north. The southwest-northeast orientation of the inlet minimizes disturbance when it is windy in the main bay. A number of good campsites make a trip in this inlet a pleasant experience. Since a boat drop-off is located in the inlet for the convenience of kayakers, it is possible to do this trip without exposure to main-bay conditions. Hazards include cold water, and occasional winds which blow—parallel to the inlet—east from the Fairweather Range.

Area Features, Background, and Tips

By 1900, ice had receded in Geikie Inlet to the extent that Shag and Tyndall coves were open, as was the bulk of the inlet west to Wood Creek. By the 1930s the entire inlet was ice-free; Geikie Glacier, grounded, was receding northwest, up its U-shaped glacial valley. At the present time, it has receded around the ridge running north from Blackthorn Peak, and is not visible from the inlet. This glacier originates from an icy labyrinth at the east edge of the massive Brady Icefield.

Geikie Inlet is 8 miles long and averages over a mile in width. Being at a right angle to the prevailing winds, the inlet is not greatly affected by air movement in the main parts of Glacier Bay. During periods of fair weather with warm temperatures, however, cold air accumulates above the ice on the east slope of the Brady Icefield. Warming in the inlet causes the air there to rise, allowing the colder air above to flow down the drainages in a rush. These sudden glacial winds arise unheralded, often blowing parallel to Geikie Inlet. Numerous, small indentations along both shores of the inlet offer protection from glacial winds, as do Tyndall and Shag coves. Yet, prevailing breezes, concentrated by Charpentier Inlet's narrow trough, can cross the low neck of intervening land, producing crosswinds in Geikie Inlet.

A tour boat, drop-off point is located on Geikie Inlet's north shore, about 1 mile from the entrance. A driftwood post set in a small rock cairn on an alder-lined beach identifies it. Check with park personnel to determine the location of the drop-off at the particular time of your trip.

An intriguing estuary lies on the north shore of Geikie Inlet 0.7 mile west of the topo survey mark MINK. You gain entrance by paddling a narrow channel (a few yards wide) that leads through a small tidal flat. Once inside, be prepared for a series of tiny bays strung end to end for a distance of several hundred yards. While a considerable current can pass through the entrance channel, you can either paddle it or line your boat.

Wood Creek, at the inlet's heel, is shown on the marine chart as possibly being navigable, luring the paddler to visit Wood Lake. Unfortunately, the creek cannot be navigated, being a jumble of alder. Although Wood Lake is an enticing 3 miles long, dragging your boat there is not worth the extreme effort. Tyndall Cove, 3 miles long, is cradled between the steep slopes of 2448' Mt. Skarn on the west, and 3274' Tlingit Peak and its ridge systems on the east. Camping is not feasible in Tyndall Cove.

Marble Mountain forms the impressive south entrance point of Geikie Inlet. This massive limestone mountain comes close to being an island rising from the sea, for only a very low, lake-studded causeway connects it to the mainland. At 3366 feet, it is the landmark around which local navigation centers. Shag Cove defines the Marble Mountain peninsula on the west, where cliffs plunge 3000 feet to water level. Camping may be possible at several locations on rocky beaches below the cliffs, depending upon the height of the tide. Since the head of Shag Cove and its entire west shore are forested, camping there is not good.

Near the west entrance point to Shag Cove are an island and an islet that form a peninsula at low tide. Good camping is possible on either. The island, 0.1 mile offshore, is edged by tidal flats. As with all island camping, be sure to carry sufficient water with you. Fresh water sources are usually not present on small islands. Another little island in Geikie Inlet is 0.3 mile offshore, between Tyndall and Shag coves. Camping is possible on this islet but surrounding mud flats can restrict access, or dictate landing during high tides. Otherwise it is an intriguing spot. Check to see if a black bear is sharing occupancy of your island before you set up camp.

Trip Description

If you are paddling this trip as a continuation of Trip 10: from Blue Mouse Cove (Map 13), paddle 3.5 miles south to the steep north point of Hugh Miller Mountain. Continue 3 miles southeast along the steep shore of 2765' Hugh Miller Mountain (Map 14). Here, an inflowing stream has created a gravel beach where you can land. From the stream, paddle 3 miles south to the entrance to Geikie Inlet at the topo survey mark FLAT. Camping is possible in a small cove 0.3 mile east of FLAT. From this cove, go 1 mile southwest to the Geikie tour boat drop-off.

This trip begins at the Geikie drop-off point, on the north shore approximately 1 mile from the inlet mouth. From the drop-off, paddle 2 miles southwest to a small but distinct sandy point, near the topo survey mark ARCH. There are campsites here. A tiny lake lies a short distance inland. Paddle 1 mile west from ARCH to an intriguing, miniature estuary inset 0.2 mile from the rest of the shoreline. Exploring is fun here if you can manage the sometimes swift current pouring out of the estuary during ebb tides. The south end of Charpentier Inlet is only 1 mile northwest across a low, alder-studded land neck.

Beyond the entrance to the small estuary, Geikie's north shore curves southwesterly in a graceful arc, adorned with mini coves, small points, and occasional shallows. Paddle 3 miles along this shore to a stream which drains the south slope of Mt. Bulky. Tidal flats line the shore around the mouth of the stream. Continue 1 mile beyond the stream, to the west side of a broad point marking the bend of the inlet. Here the shoreline is more open; camping is possible near the Geikie Glacier outwash and its tidal flats. On the north shore to the west are large gravel moraines.

Paddle parallel to the 0.7-mile-wide outwash to Geikie's cottonwood-lined south shore. Paddle 1.5 miles east to explore a cove set 0.3 mile back from the shoreline; its stream provides an outlet for an inland lake. East of this cove, you pass the survey mark DINGO and enter Wood Creek Cove. You will probably find Wood Creek a jungle of alder. After leaving Wood Creek, paddle north along the wooded shoreline for 1.5 miles. Then head 0.5 mile east to where a small peninsula with the topo survey mark KNOB projects from the shoreline. Paddle 2 miles east from KNOB to the mouth of Tyndall Cove. There are possible, yet poor, campsites near the stream at the cove's west entrance.

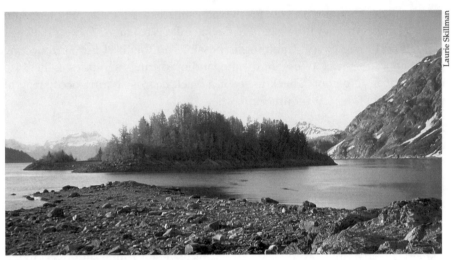

Island in Geikie Inlet

From the stream, go 2.5 miles to the head of Tyndall Cove to experience this forested, narrow fiord bordered by imposing peaks on either side. Camping at the head of the cove is, once again, possible but not ideal (14 miles from the Geikie drop-off).

From the head of Tyndall Cove, paddle 3 miles north to the east entrance at the topo survey mark BUTE. Head 2 miles east from BUTE to the entrance point of Shag Cove. Near the midpoint between Tyndall and Shag coves, a small island beckons from 0.3 mile offshore. Camping is possible there. At the west entrance to Shag Cove, a narrow peninsula with a small, wooded area at the northeast end, makes an excellent campsite (19 miles from the Geikie drop-off). Be aware that this site becomes an island at high tide. A few hundred yards to the north, is an islet with a possible campsite.

From the west point, go 2 miles southeast to the head of Shag Cove. This section treats you to the steep, wooded west shore and the precipitous, open slopes of Marble Mountain to the east. Watch for mountain goats along this section. At the head of Shag Cove, retrace your 2-mile paddle along the enticing gravel beach below Marble's steep slopes and cliffs. While there are camping possibilities in places, flat areas safely above the tidemark are scarce. Continue paddling 1.5 miles north along the west shore of Marble Mountain to its westernmost point, near the mouth of Geikie Inlet. While there are minor gravel beaches to be found in this area, I don't recommend camping because surf generated by Glacier Bay's wind waves can dampen sites close to the tideline. If you are continuing on to Trip 12, this is your turnoff point. If you are ending your trip at the tour boat pickup point in Geikie Inlet, cross the 1.5-mile-wide inlet mouth; then paddle 1 mile southwest to the pickup point (25 miles round trip).

From all appearances we were paddling on a large, inland lake. This beautiful body of water emanated calm, from the shoreline bordered by tall cottonwoods, to the high, snowy peaks that surrounded us. Geikie Inlet was casting its spell, enticing us to spend some time amid coves and estuaries. Bright sun sparkled from the surface riffles, gently backlit the cottonwoods' emerging leaves, yet glared unmercifully above 1000 feet from a remaining winter snowpack. We marvelled at the ninth straight day of sunshine, a good luck streak having its downside in the winds this weather fostered. Our paddling rate had slowed as we entered Geikie Inlet, trading the choppy, open waters of Glacier Bay for the relaxing bliss here. As usual, we began searching for the ideal campsite.

Along the shore, small flocks of harlequin and goldeneye ducks paddled out of our way. Conspicuous in May cottonwoods, bald eagles perched at respectable intervals. Rounding a point revealed a shallow cove where a large black bear busied in the intertidal area. Drifting closer, we watched as the animal smashed dozens of the barnacles carpeting the rocks. Placing a front paw on the rock, the bear leaned forward, and then with weight on its paw, twisted back and forth. Next came an industrious licking of smashed barnacles from paw and rock alike, after which the process was repeated. We drifted, 50 feet away, and watched.

The warm sun and mild conditions made us lazy. We chose a beach campsite a short distance from our barnacle-eating bear, and unloaded the kayak. A blue heron decided that the beach was too small for all of us, and scolded as it flapped away.

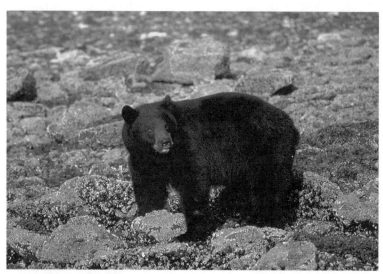

Black bear in intertidal area

A pair of black oystercatchers twittered their loud territorial call from the water's edge. As we were writing in our logs toward evening, the oystercatchers approached within a few yards of our tent. The pair then crouched, fluttered, and backed away a few quick steps, luring us to follow. This is the oystercatchers' normal routine to deflect possible enemies from their nest. So we played the game, wondering where the nest actually was. Next morning we found it. The oystercatchers had been leading us toward their two, mottled-brown eggs. Had they somehow become disoriented? We'll never know. But that pair of oystercatchers seemed to delight in approaching us during our short stay on their beach.

The next day we explored the length of Geikie Inlet to its toe and heel. Paddling back toward the mouth, we explored narrow, fiord-like Tyndall Cove. Evening found us in Shag Cove near the inlet mouth. Mountain goats grazed unhurriedly on precipitous Marble Mountain's narrow ledges. The elevated tip of a narrow peninsula where we camped became an island later at high tide. A black bear hurriedly vacated the wooded, house-sized point as we approached our intended campsite. The bear eyed us, then agilely conveyed its bulk past us and into the woods.

It is after 10:00 P.M., and we are still too exhausted to sleep. From the nearby forest comes the deep booming of a male grouse. A flock of Canada geese passes overhead, adding its wind-instrument section to the grouse's bass. Then, unbelievably, the soft song of a warbler fills in the strings. Before the symphony ends, we are asleep.

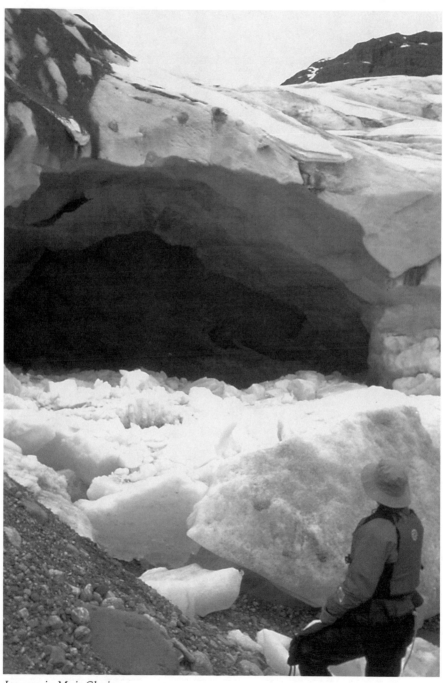

Ice cave in Muir Glacier

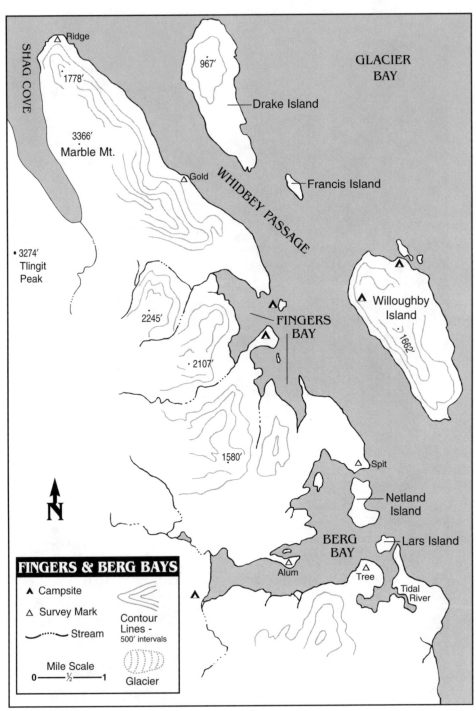

SHAG COVE

△ Ridge

·1778'

3366'
Marble Mt.

GLACIER
BAY

967'

Drake Island

△Gold

WHIDBEY PASSAGE

Francis Island

·3274'
Tlingit
Peak

·2245'

·2107'

𐤠

FINGERS
BAY

Willoughby
Island

·1662'

1580'

N

△ Spit

Netland
Island

Lars Island

BERG BAY

Alum

△
Tree

Tidal
River

FINGERS & BERG BAYS

🔺 Campsite

△ Survey Mark

······ Stream

Contour
Lines -
500' intervals

Glacier

Mile Scale
0 —— ½ —— 1

MAP 15

Chapter 16

TRIP 12 **FINGERS AND BERG BAYS FROM GEIKIE INLET**

Trip Details

Distance:	40 miles RT from Geikie Inlet drop-off
	45 miles from Geikie drop-off to Bartlett Cove
Time:	5-6 days
Rating:	Moderate to Difficult
Maps:	NOAA chart 17318; USGS Topos: Mt. Fairweather (C-1), (C-2), & (D-2); Juneau (C-6)

Summary and Highlights

Fingers and Berg bays offer conditions much like those in the Beardslee Islands, both in terms of protected water, and the maturation of the forest there. These two bays offer an environment much less harsh than that which is found in the bays and inlets farther north. Because of good water clarity, intertidal life as well as marine bottom dwellers are plentiful in this area. Many shallows in these two bays present virtual aquariums for the kayaking naturalist. Also of interest is the impressive tidal river located 0.5 mile southeast just inside the south entrance of Berg Bay. Although the water here is several degrees warmer than that at the north end of Glacier Bay, it is still a hazard for kayakers. If you didn't have to paddle 9 miles each way through Whidbey Passage, this trip would be rated "easy." The possibility of wind and waves makes this a stretch which must be paddled with caution and when conditions are calm.

Area Features, Background, and Tips

Fingers and Berg bays became ice-free at about the same time as the Beardslee Island group, in the early to mid-1800s. As a result, the establishment of forests has progressed for over 150 years, enabling the growth of mature spruce and cottonwood, some 2 feet in diameter, or greater. Both bays have large expanses of shallow water; their deepest spot is just over 200 feet, while mid-channel depths in Glacier Bay waterways near the bays average over 300 feet. As in other bays and inlets, glacial deposits of till, alluvium and silt altered the shoreline and bottom contours. One noticeable difference from other estuaries, with the glaciers far receded over many intervening years, is the lack of recent silt deposition. Sizable portions of the bottom are clean rock and gravel. Clean marine environments attract bottom dwellers such as sea stars, anemones, urchins, mollusks, and arthropods. Many specimens present brilliant coloration, making some areas with dense colonies of various species appear kaleidoscopic.

The same water clarity which enables the viewing of bottom dwellers also entices various anadromous fish species. While a few streams in upper Glacier Bay are used for spawning by salmon and trout, in the lower bay, a greater number of streams provide these fish with spawning beds. In Fingers Bay, and especially Berg Bay, the clear streams are home to coho and sockeye salmon; Dolly Varden and cutthroat trout. King, the largest of the salmon, visit Berg Bay.

Spawning salmon mean a rich food source for many animals. Most noticeable are the bears. Both brown and black bears congregate around salmon streams during spawning runs to feed on healthy fish, or spawned-out carcasses. Seals and other animals such as coyotes, foxes, otter, and mink also feed on carcasses. Bald eagles and ravens make use of this important food supply.

Many biologists believe that the only difference between the inland, or mountain, grizzly and the larger coastal brown bear is the presence of the rich, marine food source. Generous amounts of fat and protein are available to bears living on the coast from anadromous fish, and intertidal sources. By contrast, inland grizzlies must work much harder to secure food. This disparity in their food supply may account for the marked difference in the bears' average sizes.

A short distance beyond the north end of Fingers Bay, the long, elevated spine of Marble Mountain rises abruptly from a flat, wooded fore-plain. The trailing ridges of Tlingit Peak west of the bay also follow this pattern. Other mountains in the vicinity rarely reach 2500 feet, mere foothills compared to Glacier Bay's lofty, northern peaks. West of Berg Bay the Fairweather Range trails off to the south; with Brady Glacier in between, it is some 20 miles distant.

Observing the trees here makes understanding the concept of an "even-age stand" easy. Since all members of each species began life at about the same time, they are approximately the same height. Consequently, the forest around Fingers and Berg bays appears to have been trimmed to a uniform height.

The land here is still rising, at nearly the same rate as in the Beardslee Islands. Lars Island, at the south entrance to Berg Bay, is essentially a peninsula now, except at the highest tides. The north passage into Berg, around the north end of Netland Island, is also a tidal flat at low water. The main channel, between Netland and Lars Islands, is shallow and subject to strong, though not particularly dangerous, currents during peak flows. Both bays offer sheltered water regardless of wind direction. Because of the close proximity to Icy Straight and its moist environment, fog may be encountered, particularly during periods when the weather is clear in the upper portions of the bay. Campsites are easy to find. Uplifting has raised many beaches above the high tidemark.

Just inside the southeast passage into Berg Bay is a small estuary with a surface area slightly less than 1 square mile. This body of water becomes isolated on ebb tides; the water level in Berg Bay drops faster than the water can

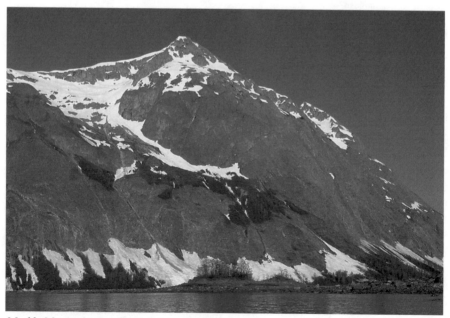

Marble Mountain guards the entrance to Geikie Inlet

drain out of the estuary's narrow, shallow channel. The result is a roaring, 0.2-mile-long, white-water river with rocks and severe rapids in the narrow channel. In the estuary above, the water level may be several feet higher than in Berg Bay. Drainage continues until the water level in the estuary falls to the level of the channel bottom, or until the rising tide equalizes water levels somewhat higher. During full flow the sound of the rapids can be heard for miles.

Trip Description

You may embark on Trip 12 from the west point of Marble Mountain as a continuation of Trip 11. In this case, continue 1 mile northeast to the topo survey mark RIDGE. The trip description assumes you are starting from the tour boat drop-off in Geikie Inlet, and mileage begins there. From the drop-off paddle 1 mile northeast to the inlet mouth; choose fair weather for your 1.5-mile crossing southeast to RIDGE at the north tip of Marble Mountain. Continue southeast along the flank of Marble Mtn. (Map 15). As a matter of fact, the next 7 miles is actually a paddle to get around the huge bulk of this 3366' mountain. The shoreline offers little protection.

A small indentation with a gravel beach offers shelter and emergency camping 0.5 mile south of RIDGE. From here paddle 3 miles south to a stream draining the west slope of Marble Mountain. This section of shoreline is rough, with precipitous, open slopes, gradually becoming less steep, but forested down to the water. A close inspection could reveal one or two precarious landing sites along this stretch, depending upon the wind and swell directions. Continue 0.7 mile southeast to a shallow indentation north of the point at topo survey mark GOLD. This site provides a good haul-out with fair camping unless there are severe swells from the north. Paddle 3 miles southeast from here to the entrance to Fingers Bay. This stretch offers few, if any, good haul-outs.

At the entrance, turn west into Fingers Bay after passing several rounded islands which can become the points of low-lying peninsulas at lower tides. The 300-yard-long island has good camping at a point on its west side. Drinking water here must come from a stream which enters at the north end of Fingers Bay. Once inside the bay, paddle 1 mile to the north end, where you can collect water from the inflow stream. Then follow the shoreline 1.5 miles to the small bay just north of the central peninsula. There are extensive tidal flats here. Leave the bay and continue 1 mile around the head of the peninsula to its south shore, where there are good campsites with a gravel beach. Exploring all the coves of the south portion of Fingers Bay from here is a pleasant 2-mile paddle that takes you to the south entrance point of the bay.

Leaving Fingers Bay, go 2 miles southeast around the headland between Fingers and Berg bays. If the water is not too low, you can enter Berg Bay around the point with the topo survey mark SPIT. Even if the channel is not fully passable, enter it anyway to look at the marine animals living in the intertidal area there. If the channel is dry, circumnavigate Netland Island and come in through the main entrance. The best campsites are found on the west side of the island. From the north channel, it is 1 mile to the north end of the bay. Just west of there, a clear stream enters. Head south and paddle 2 miles along the west shore of Berg Bay. There are islands and small coves to explore along this stretch, ending at the long peninsula bearing the topo survey mark ALUM. From ALUM, turn west and paddle 2 miles to the head of the bay (22 miles from the Geikie drop-off). Good camping is available here on a bench back from the water, but tidal flats demand that you be careful where you tie your boat. Clear streams enter the bay at the west end. If salmon are in the streams, don't camp here; find yourself a spot well away from the bears' dinner table.

From the streams, go 3 miles east along the south shore to a narrow point with the topo survey mark TREE, which is surrounded by tidal flats. Lars Island, which appears like a peninsula, lies 0.3 mile northeast of this point. A few hundred yards east of TREE is a sizable tidal river, often visually and audibly apparent, that runs when water is leaving the estuary on the ebb tide. You won't be able to paddle against the current in this river, and going with it becomes a whitewater slalom between impossible rocks. At high tide, the saltwater rapids disappear. You can paddle through at high tide's slack water in either direction, or north from the estuary when the ebb is just beginning. Exploring the 1.5-mile-long estuary is fun, but be very cautious here.

Go 1 mile northeast from the tidal river to the main entrance to Berg Bay at the south end of Netland Island (26 miles from the Geikie drop-off). From Netland Island, paddle north-northwest along the shore to the beginning point at the Geikie pickup. The pickup point is 14 miles distant, if you don't take any side trips on your return trip (40 miles round trip).

* * * *

Should you not wish to paddle back to Geikie Inlet but prefer instead to return to park headquarters in Bartlett Cove, you will need to cross Glacier Bay. Strawberry Island looks enticingly near at hand—a 2.5-mile crossing at most—but don't even think about it. Sitakaday Narrows intervenes, and this channel is notorious for swift currents, whirlpools, and tiderips. All the tides within Glacier Bay flow in and out through Sitakaday Narrows.

To begin the 19-mile-long route back to park headquarters from Netland Island, paddle 4 miles north to the north channel in to Fingers Bay. Carefully select your departure time with an eye to both weather and current, then make the 1-mile crossing to the north end of Willoughby Island. Early mornings are often the best time for crossing. Camping on Willoughby Island is

possible on the west side, 1 mile south of the north end, and at several locations among coves and islets at the northeast end. Should fast-flowing currents or rising winds become a concern, you can haul out on the island and
wait for improvements.

From Willoughby Island's east side, paddle 3 miles due east across open
water to the vicinity of Flapjack Island and its extensive tidal flats. This is by
far the longest open-water paddle described in this book, and you should be
cautious of winds and currents. Flapjack is one of the Beardslee Islands, and
from here to Bartlett Cove is an easy, 9-mile paddle. Once in the Beardslees
you can follow the Trip 1 route back to Bartlett Cove.

⊷ ⊨◊⊨ ⊶

*Southbound through Whidbey Passage, our bow gurgling on the surface as the
early morning breeze boosted our speed, we were catching up fast with a pod of
humpbacks. The whales were diving deep in 300 feet of water, surfacing every few
minutes. The vapor of their breath hung in the air, then slowly disappeared. Within
a few hundred yards, we stopped paddling and drifted, watching the behemoths.
Since their course led into the main channel north of Willoughby Island, we part-
ed company, heading for two picturesque, southwestern bays.*

*Contrasting with the wind-driven swells of the channel, only ripples scored the
surface inside Fingers Bay. We paddled into the north half, skirting a flock of*

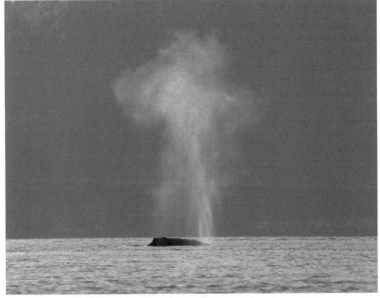

Humpback whale spouting near Willoughby Island

white-front geese which eyed us suspiciously. Two ravens—reveling in flight—swooped and rolled in unison before gliding to shore; on landing, they scolded us with a call common to wilderness and suburbia alike. We obliged by scooting elsewhere, leaving the ravens to their beach. We reentered Whidbey Passage. Visibility to the south was diminishing, and within minutes wisps of fog obscured all except the near shore.

Cutting through the dense fog, we turned into Berg Bay at its north channel, and found ourselves above an unbelievable tidal aquarium. Beneath the clear water a few feet offshore, dozens of vari-colored sea stars and urchins patterned and populated the bottom. Hundreds of water spouts rising from a nearby beach exposed at low tide amazed us on landing. Somewhat dazed, we stepped ashore only to be sprinkled by the spouting clams. The almost comical, mad cacophony of a multiclam fountain entertained us as we ate brunch.

The deafening sound of rushing water drew us to southeast Berg Bay just as the fog lifted. A rushing, turbulent tidal river spilled out and into Berg Bay from the elevated pool of a sizable estuary. These ebb-tide rapids and drops would have severely tested our boating abilities, had we been inclined to challenge them. The current generated caused riffles and tiderips visible hundreds of yards out into the bay. While we watched the tidal river from shore, a large black bear emerged noisily from a nearby spruce thicket, and stood looking directly at us. This threatening behavior made us uneasy, and it was a minute or two before the bear yielded to verbal persuasion and lumbered away.

Back in our kayak, we spent a while adjusting to the overall character of Berg Bay. Meanwhile, sun had superseded fog, and warmed us. We took a last look westward, where the modest ridges of the Fairweathers trailed away to the south. With the roar of tidal rapids in our ears, we turned and paddled slowly toward the inlet mouth, with eyes peeled on the marine aquarium beneath us. Then our kayak was bobbing rhythmically in wind waves as we headed north.

Appendix 1—Services, Sources, and Tips

General Information

Glacier Bay National Park and Reserve, P.O. Box 140, Gustavus, AK 99826-0140, (907) 697-2230.

Gustavus Visitor Association, P.O. Box 167, Gustavus, AK 99826.

Transportation

Alaska Marine Highway System, P.O. Box 25535, Juneau, AK 99802-5535, (800) 642-0066. Ferry for passengers, vehicles and kayaks from Bellingham, WA to Juneau, AK.

Glacier Bay Tours & Cruises, 520 Pike St., Suite 1400, Seattle, WA 98101, (800) 451-5925. Passenger catamaran which carries kayaks from Juneau, AK to Gustavus, AK.

Alaska Airlines, (800) 426-0333. Air transportation from Seattle, WA and other northwest cities to Juneau, AK. Collapsible kayaks can usually be accommodated on commercial airlines.

Air Excursions, P.O. Box 16, Gustavus, AK 99826, (907) 697-2375. Scheduled and chartered air transportation from Juneau, AK to Gustavus, AK. Cannot transport rigid kayaks, but can usually accommodate collapsible boats when notified ahead.

Frontier Air, P.O. Box 1, Gustavus, AK 99826, (907) 697-2386. Scheduled and chartered air transportation from Juneau, AK to Gustavus, AK. Cannot transport rigid kayaks, but can usually accommodate collapsible boats when notified ahead.

Ground Transportation

Glacier Bay Lodge, P.O. Box 199, Gustavus, AK 99826, (907) 697-2225. Bus from lodge to Gustavus, airport, and pier.

TLC Taxi, P.O. Box 103, Gustavus, AK 99806, (907) 697-2239. On-call transportation from Gustavus airport to park headquarters. Have rack for kayak transport.

Camping

The Park Service provides a free walk-in campground near the headquarters at Bartlett Cove.

Up-Bay Drop-off, Tour Boat, Lodging

Glacier Bay Lodge, P.O. Box 199, Gustavus, AK 99826, (800) 451-5952. This concessionaire provides the valuable drop-off service that enables many kayakers to visit the heart of Glacier Bay during a short stay. Lodging is available in several classes. In addition to the traditional lodge, a laundromat, showers, and dormitories cater to the independent paddler. The lodge features a restaurant, a varied menu, and a view of Bartlett Cove.

Kayak Outfitters

Alaska Discovery, 5449-4K Shaune Drive, Juneau, AK 99801, (800) 586-1911. Group kayak trips in Glacier Bay.

Spirit Walker Expeditions, P.O. Box 240, Gustavus, AK 99826, (800) 529-2537. Group kayak trips in Glacier Bay.

Kayak Rentals

Glacier Bay Lodge, P.O. Box 199, Gustavus, AK 99826 (800) 451-5952. Rental of single and double kayaks and paddles.

Sea Otter Kayaks, P.O. Box 228, Gustavus, AK 99826 (907) 697-3007. Rental of single and double kayaks and paddles.

Charter Boats

Mystic Sea Charters, P.O. Box 324, Gustavus, AK 99826, (888) 699-8422. Whale watching, fishing, sightseeing. Owners Aaron & Erin Bohlke live in Gustavus year round.

Bear-Resistant Containers

Containers are provided without charge by the Park Service. Should you wish to purchase one or more containers for use elsewhere, they are available from:

Alaska Natural History Association, P.O. Box 140, Gustavus, AK 99826, (907) 697-2635. The Association also stocks and sells a number of excellent books specific to Glacier Bay.

Map Sources

USGS Topographical maps are available from the following sources:

Western Distribution Branch, U.S. Geological Survey, Box 25286, Federal Center, Denver, CO 80225. Maps, keys, and symbol explanation are also available from this federal government agency.

Powers Elevation Co., (303) 321-2217. USGS Topos, NOAA charts. They are near the USGS office in Denver, CO, and can supply any USGS map. Credit card orders.

Map Centre, Inc., 2611 University Ave., San Diego, CA 92104-3830, (619) 291-3830. USGS Topos, NOAA charts, other maps. Credit card orders.

The Map Center, 2440 Bancroft Way, Berkeley, CA 94704, (510) 841-MAPS (841-6277). USGS Topos, NOAA charts. Credit card orders.

Equipment Tips

Kayaks. Most manufacturers produce well-made and well-designed boats. For touring Glacier Bay, whether single or double, a kayak should be designed primarily as a sea kayak, and possess a rudder. Sea kayaks should have sufficient volume to provide adequate storage space for gear and supplies. Designs that present unnecessarily elevated bows to the wind should be avoided. Sit-upon boats are not appropriate, nor are kayaks designed primarily for whitewater use. Construction materials, if good quality, make little difference.

Paddles. You will be using that paddle all day long, day after day. Weight and balance are very important factors. Most paddles are extremely strong. Be sure your paddle is sufficiently long that you do not have to adjust your stroke for the paddle to clear your gunwales. Carry an extra, 2-piece paddle lashed on deck as a spare.

Safety Gear. Once away from Bartlett Cove you are on your own, so make sure your PFD, spray skirt, paddle float, and bilge pump are correctly designed and honestly made. What looks good in the showroom doesn't necessarily work well under adverse conditions. Practice your safety maneuvers.

Miscellaneous tips. Consider using a transparent vinyl map case, lashed under your deck bungees, for charts, folded to expose the area being paddled. Coat charts with water-based polyurethane water proofing before you leave. Make sure your deck compass swings freely, and has no air bubbles.

A pair of binoculars is ideal for viewing wildlife, and making out distant navigation features. The pair we used was an excellent, 8-power compact binocular by Swarovski, the only truly waterproof glass we could find. Salt water never bothered the binoculars even when we kept them on deck.

For transporting a rigid boat, which invariably will contain gear, we found that a dolly was indispensable. A strong, folding unit such as that designed by Primex, is ideal. The lightweight aluminum frame with pneumatic tires handled our 20' boat with ease, even when we wheeled it several miles along roadways.

Appendix 2—Recommended Reading

About Glacier Bay

National Park Service, *Glacier Bay, A Guide to Glacier Bay National Park and Preserve, Alaska*, Handbook 123, 1983.

Jettmar, *Alaska's Glacier Bay: A Traveller's Guide*, Alaska Northwest Books, 1997.

Heacox, Kim, *Boating in Glacier Bay National Park & Preserve*, Alaska Natural History Association, 1987.

Graef, Kris, *The Alaska Wilderness Guide*, Vernon Publications, Inc., 1993.

Flora & Fauna

Russo, Ron and Olhausen, Pam, *Pacific Intertidal Life*, Nature Study Guild, 1981.

Meinkoth, Norman A., *National Audubon Society Field Guide to North American Seashore Creatures*, Alfred A. Knopf, 1995.

Armstrong, Robert H., *Guide To The Birds Of Alaska*, Alaska Northwest Publishing, 1986.

Caldwell, David K., *National Audubon Society Field Guide to North American Fishes, Whales & Dolphins*, Alfred A. Knopf, 1988.

Whitaker, John O. Jr., *The Audubon Society Field Guide to North American Mammals*, Alfred A. Knopf, 1988.

Wheat, Ellen (ed.), *The Alaska-Yukon Wild Flowers Guide*, Alaska Northwest Publishing Company, 1988.

Viereck, Les, *Alaska Trees and Shrubs*, University of Alaska Press, 1986.

Kayaking

Jettmar, Karen, *The Alaska River Guide*, Alaska Northwest Books, 1993.

Hutchinson, Derek C., *Derek C. Hutchinson's Guide to Expedition Kayaking on Sea & Open Water*, The Globe Pequot Press, 1990.

Hutchinson, Derek C., *The Complete Book Of Sea Kayaking*, The Globe Pequot Press, 1994.

Keating, W. R., *Survival in Cold Water*, Blackwell Scientific Publishers, 1969.

Burch, David, *Fundamentals of Kayak Navigation*, Globe Pequot Press, 1987.

General Outdoors

Wilkerson, James A., M.D., *Medicine for Mountaineering*, The Mountaineers Books, 1985.

Forgey, William W., *Wilderness Medicine*, ICS Books, 1987.

Darvill, Fred T., Jr., M.D., *Mountaineering Medicine*, 14th ed., Wilderness Press, 1998.

Index

Kayaking on open water entails unavoidable risk that every kayaker assumes and must be aware of and respect. The fact that a trip is described in this book is not a representation that it will be safe for you. Kayaking trips vary greatly in difficulty and in the degree of conditioning and skill one needs to enjoy them safely. On some trips the area may have changed or conditions may have deteriorated since the descriptions were written. Trip conditions change even from day to day, owing to weather and other factors. A trip that is safe on a calm day or for a highly conditioned, experienced, properly equipped kayaker may be completely unsafe for someone else or unsafe under adverse weather conditions.

You can minimize your risks on the water by being knowledgeable, prepared and alert. There is not space in this book for a general treatise on safety on the water, but there are a number of good books and instruction courses on the subject and you should take advantage of them to increase your knowledge. Just as important, you should always be aware of your own limitations and of conditions existing when and where you are kayaking. If conditions are dangerous, or if you're not prepared to deal with them safely, choose a different trip, or don't go at all. It's better to have wasted a drive than to be the subject of a rescue. These warnings are not intended to scare you off the water. However, one element of the beauty, freedom and excitement of kayaking is the presence of risks that do not confront us at home. When you kayak you assume those risks. They can be met safely, but only if you exercise your own independent judgement and common sense. The author and the publisher of this book disclaim any liability or loss resulting from the use of this book.

Grab your paddle
and put in with our new
Adventure Kayaking series...

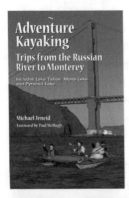

Adventure Kayaking: Trips from the Russian River to Monterey

Michael Jeneid

Explore 150 miles of beautiful lagoons, bays, and esteros of the Central California coastline from the Russian River to Monterey with this book's 24 day trips for kayak.

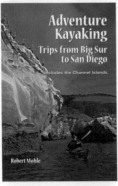

Adventure Kayaking: Trips from Big Sur to San Diego

Robert Mohle

This book has over 50 trips along the Southern California coastline. Paddle along the magnificent coast of Big Sur, among the scenic Channel Islands, and past the sparkling beaches of northern San Diego county.

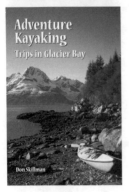

Adventure Kayaking: Trips in Glacier Bay

Don Skillman

Enjoy the deep blue glacial waters of Southeast Alaska by paddle! This book covers over 300 miles of trips in and around Glacier Bay and Glacier Bay National Park.

For more information on these and other **Wilderness Press** titles, contact us at *(800) 443-7227* or *mail@wildernesspress.com*